Awakening Athena

Awakening Athena

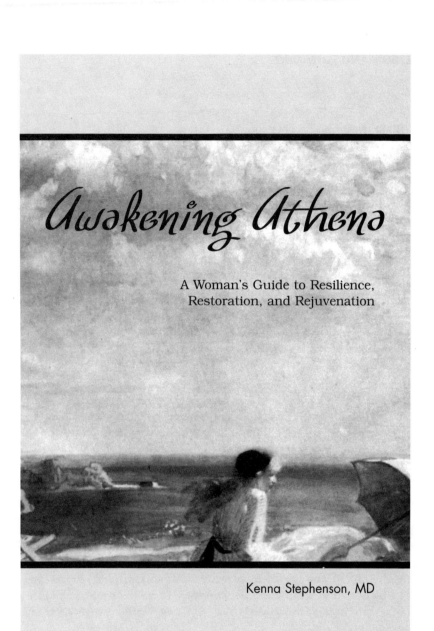

A Woman's Guide to Resilience,
Restoration, and Rejuvenation

Kenna Stephenson, MD

Health, Heart & Mind Institute • Tyler, Texas

Awakening Athena

Health, Heart & Mind Institute — Tyler, Texas

Published by Health, Heart & Mind Institute, 2702 East 5th St, #362, Tyler, TX 75701

ISBN 0-9758681-0-1

Printed in the United States of America

Design by Karin Wilson, Wild Woman Design; www.WildWomanDesign.com and Katie Baird, Loose Ends; www.LooseEnds.net

Kenna Stephenson, MD, does not receive remuneration for the endorsements of products, devices, books, videos, services, individuals, or organizations. Corporations or companies providing the products mentioned in *Awakening Athena* do not endorse that book or necessarily agree with its content.

The opinions expressed in *Awakening Athena* are those of Dr. Stephenson, and the information therein is based on both the author's clinical experience and a thorough review of the medical literature. The information in this book is not intended to serve as a substitute for diagnosis, medical advice, or treatment by a licensed clinician. Each patient's medical and psychologic needs are unique, and readers are advised not to change their current treatment without consulting their physician or healthcare professional. The author and publisher accept no liability associated with the use of the information in *Awakening Athena*.

Every effort has been made to protect the confidentiality of each patient presented in the case histories. However, for clinical accuracy and educational purposes, the core content and patient responses to specific therapies have not been altered. Patients who are identified by name have given their written consent for such identification.

To my husband, Douglas, who has given me encouragement and hope

To my children, who have given me life's greatest joy

To my mother, Julia Beth, who has loved me always and whose belief in me has never faltered

Acknowledgements

It has been a sacred experience to have cared for the patients who are anonymous contributors to this book. The stories shared in *Awakening Athena* are those of many girls and women whom I have known professionally and personally during the last 20 years. The privilege of sharing their pain, struggle, trauma, hope, and transformation has been a humbling experience. It is my hope that by giving voice to the physical, emotional, and spiritual recovery of the patients profiled here, *Awakening Athena* will be a comfort and inspiration to others. To all of those women, thank you.

The contribution of my editor, Jane Vail, has been invaluable. Her skillful editing through several drafts, her mature perspective, and her gentle direction guided and grounded me when I felt overwhelmed in the unknown territory of writing a book. Her advice, patience, and encouragement through many discussions of the book's purpose and the readers' needs brought forth a manuscript that exudes an elegance, passion, and truth that could not have been achieved without her tireless attention.

My design team, Katie Baird at Loose Ends and Karin Wilson of Wild Woman Design, have provided the gifts of sensitive hands, design perspective, and valuable advice in bringing the manuscript to life. I am also grateful for the assistance of Jim Paoletti, RPh, who reviewed the formulary for compounded medications that is featured in Chapter 6.

Several of my teachers and senior colleagues in medicine, who have inspired me and influenced my practice and research, deserve recognition and thanks: Duane Andrews, MD; Ben Bridges, MD; Ralph Anderson, MD; James Dumbauld, DO; Al Prause, MD; Thomas Tenner, PhD; and Hal Werner, MD.

Other friends who participated in the development of *Awakening Athena* should be recognized for their contributions as well. They offered assistance with home and family needs, meal preparation, home repair and maintenance, car repair, child care, and transportation. They provided emotional support and made sure that I occasionally stopped writing and had some fun! Special thanks to Hubert and Janet A, Don and Mara B, Megan B, Kevin and Kathy D, Lucy L, Emily L, Todd and Missy N, Jennifer P, Shawn P, Guy and Barbara P, Carol P, Karin S, Pam S, Lisa S, Larry and Janice S, and John and Waynie S. Mary C, Sherry R, and Charli T were instrumental in the early development of this book by providing personal and professional support.

Contents

Foreword

I have had the privilege of caring for thousands of women patients during my career as a physician. They have been my greatest teachers. My practice, in return, supports Dr. Carl Jung's theory that **all** women can transform themselves to their benefit by improving their health and well-being. Even our most traumatic experiences do not sentence us to a life of misery and failure. The power to change and overcome is within us all.

Resilience, wisdom, compassion, and courage have been associated with the essential female self, the feminine archetype, since antiquity. In contemporary American society, women have an urgent need to awaken within themselves the archetype of Athena, the Greek goddess of wisdom, war, and healing. Athena lived and excelled in a patriarchal society. She, like many of my women patients, was born into conflict. According to tradition, Athena was denied infancy, childhood, and maternal nurturing. She sprang, fully grown and fully clothed in protective armor, from the head of her father, Zeus. Athena was despised by her stepmother and became the target of her half-siblings' envy. She was a victim of deceit, personal attacks, and abuse. In spite of those challenges, she used practical thinking, intelligence, skill, courage, and reason to save herself and those she loved from defeat and injustice. She had a strong sense of self-worth, and she achieved altruistic goals without self-sacrifice. She maneuvered herself confidently and effectively in a male-dominated culture and in society at large.

Athena achieved her success by developing skills that can be used today by any woman willing to pay the psychic cost of transforming herself and her world. It is my hope that the suggestions in this book will help that effort. The practices that I recommend are readily available and affordable, and they offer many benefits. I appeal to all women to awaken Athena in themselves and to join me in seeking wisdom and self-healing.

Chapter I
Taking Control of Your Health

Athena was the Greek goddess of war and wisdom. In battle, she used her intellect and imagination in strategic planning to bring victory. This chapter is dedicated to Joan Furey, who in 1994 was appointed the first director of the Center for Women Veterans in the US Department of Veterans Affairs. As a young woman, Joan awakened her Athena archetype when she volunteered to serve our country during wartime as an Army nurse in Vietnam. Like Athena, she embodied the Army nurse motto: Ready, caring, proud. Since her retirement from the military, Joan has battled tirelessly on behalf of US women veterans on many fronts: to ensure that they receive services and benefits equal to those bestowed on male veterans, to create awareness of gender-specific health care and issues unique to women veterans, and to include women veterans in all veterans programs, including medical research.

The Effects of Gender-Biased Treatment

Gender bias in American medical care exists. As a result, many physicians and their women patients have journeyed down the wrong path of diagnosis and treatment. Gender disparity is also evident in medical research and in the types of therapy provided to men and women. For example, although cardiovascular disease kills 43,000 more American women than men each year, cardiovascular research has been conducted almost exclusively in men, and most cardiac procedures (thrombolysis, catheterization, angioplasty, bypass surgery, stenting) are performed in men.[1-4]

In 2003, researchers at the Mayo Clinic surveyed 204 women in several regions of the United States who were hospitalized for chest pain and were subsequently discharged with a diagnosis of heart disease.[5] Fifty-two percent of the respondents reported dissatisfaction with their physicians. Some women had been treated with condescension or abruptness; others had been wrongly diagnosed and their symptoms of cardiac disease had been attributed initially to panic disorder, the effects of psychologic stress, or hypochondria. In the United States, the gender bias in treatment for various diseases is related to multiple factors, but women patients *can* be proactive about their own health care without waiting for support from the research and medical communities.

Before 1990, almost all research trials for new drugs were performed solely in men. Women were excluded from participation in such studies because the "aberrations" of menstruation, menopause, pregnancy, or breast-feeding were thought to skew results. Because of that exclusion, women patients now receive many drugs tested in and approved as safe for men, although gender-specific physiologic differences can affect the response to treatment. Unfortunately, drug-related adverse effects that occur only in women are often discounted by physicians.

In 1992, the Office on Women's Health was established in the US Department of Health and Human Services as "the government's champion and focal point for women's health issues."[6] That office, in conjunction with various women's consumer groups such as the Society for the Advancement of Women's Health Research, has demanded more rigorous research of women's health issues, the inclusion of women of all ages and ethnic groups in research studies, and federal laws mandating that the Food and Drug Administration (FDA) include women (even menstruating women) in all phases of research on new drugs designed to treat both men and women. Over the last decade, these efforts have generated research studies illuminating gender-distinct differences in brain and cardiac function, pain pathways, and the response to emotional stress.[1-4,7-17] If the results from such research are regarded seriously, diagnostic testing and therapies better designed to treat female patients will be made available. Until that time (and as a general rule as well), women must *insist* that their physicians respond appropriately if treatment seems ineffective or adverse effects occur.

The "Premrose Path"

In the past, many prescribing practices for American women were based on less-than-scientific study. Between 1949 and 2002, much of the available drug therapy for perimenopausal and menopausal women was dictated more by economics, marketing, and advertising than by the scientific evidence of safety for the patient. For example, Premarin (conjugated equine estrogens derived from the urine of pregnant mares) and Prempro (a combination of Premarin plus medroxyprogesterone acetate, which is a synthetic progestin) were long considered standard treatment for menopausal symptoms. Because Premarin is derived from an animal source, its molecular structure is different from that of the estrogen produced by the human body. In my clinical opinion, that difference contributes to the likelihood of adverse effects. Premarin has been widely prescribed for more than 50 years, and Prempro, for more than 30. As recently as last year, physicians told their female patients that those hormones provided protection against heart disease, osteoporosis, and Alzheimer's disease. However, the results of the recent National Institutes of Health (NIH) Women's Health Initiative (WHI) debunked most health benefits attributed to those drugs.[18]

Results of the WHI: Reconsidering Hormone Replacement

The WHI trials were designed to assess the safety and efficacy of hormone replacement therapy (HRT) in healthy postmenopausal women. Study participants with a uterus received estrogen-plus-progestin (Prempro), and those without a uterus received estrogen alone (Premarin, which is derived from the urine of pregnant mares). Both trials were terminated early (the Prempro trial in 2002 and the Premarin trial in 2004) because the health risks of treatment outweighed the benefit of a decreased incidence of osteoporotic fractures. The trials showed that in postmenopausal women with a uterus, treatment with estrogen-plus-progestin increased the risk of invasive breast cancer, coronary heart disease, stroke, and pulmonary embolism. In postmenopausal women without a uterus, treatment with estrogen alone had no effect on coronary heart disease risk but increased the risk of stroke and significantly increased the risk of deep vein thrombosis. Those results shocked the medical community. Unfortunately, many American women had received such therapy for decades.

Even before the WHI results were released, I was concerned about the effects of HRT in postmenopausal women. In 1998, I wrote a medical journal article emphasizing 2 issues: that women were advised to take HRT to prevent osteoporosis, heart attack, or Alzheimer's disease without being told of the treatment-related risk of breast cancer and that no compelling research supported the use of HRT in healthy postmenopausal women.[19] My opinion was in the minority, but other physicians, including HRT experts John Lee, MD, and Christiane Northrup, MD, expressed similar concerns based on logic and reason (the "voice of Athena" on which this book is based).

The early termination of the WHI Prempro trial in 2002 was a wake-up call for many women receiving that therapy. In spite of those results, however, the estimated total number of US prescriptions for HRT (most of which were for Premarin or Prempro) written in 2003 was *57 million*.[20] It is clear that many women remain tangled in a web of patriarchal medicine in which irrefutable medical data are ignored.

I believe that compounded bioidentical hormone replacement therapy (BHRT), in which hormones structurally identical to those produced by the human body are used (see Chapter 6), is a safer option for women with severe perimenopausal or menopausal symptoms. Unfortunately, BHRT is greatly underutilized.

The Benefits of Gender-Specific Care

Women seeking health care in the United States today should choose a physician who practices gender-specific care: a doctor who has clinical skill in treating men and women and equal respect for both. I believe that the following 6 principles are essential to ensuring excellence in health care and a good physician-patient relationship. If applied to biomedical research, education, and patient outcome, they can minimize the gender gap in American medical treatment.

Physicians Must Treat All Patients with Respect and Compassion

My women patients have shared countless examples of being treated disrespectfully by physicians when they attempt to discuss their health concerns. One patient said that she was told by her doctor, "If Prempro is good enough for my wife and mother, then it's good enough for my patients." He refused to listen to her concerns about the risks of treatment. In answer to a question, another patient's doctor said in a hostile tone, "When you go to medical school, do a residency, and have as many diplomas on the wall as I do, then you can join in a discussion about your prescription for hormones." Recently a woman friend revealed that in response to her request for her medical test results, her doctor said, "If I gave them to you, you wouldn't understand them."

Mary C. P. Jacobi, MD, (1842 – 1906) was one of the first American female physicians. Throughout her career, Dr. Jacobi taught that compassion and pure science are equally important in the practice of medicine.[21] To protect their health and well-being, women patients today must demand both clinical excellence and compassionate health care from their physicians.

Patients Must Be Empowered to Take Charge of Their Health

This principle pertains more to the actions of the patient than to those of the physician. Each patient must make lifestyle choices that create better health. Physicians cannot undo the damage created by weeks of poor nutrition, lack of exercise, or toxic relationships simply by writing a prescription. Each woman must act as her own best advocate for staying healthy.

Years ago, I began providing my patients with a copy of their medical and laboratory test results. A printout of test results is an instant, tangible record of health that can be readily referred to, if necessary. Seeing that information in writing somehow makes it more real and motivates many patients to take a more active role in their own health care.

One of my patients was told adamantly by her former doctor that she had cancer, and she was sent for therapy to a cancer treatment facility in another city. She underwent a series of examinations at that hospital, and her disease was correctly identified as benign. Her relief was immense, but she had already been severely affected by the first diagnosis. After that experience, she became aggressively proactive about her own health care. She tape-recorded every visit to her physicians and assertively demanded photocopies of her prescriptions and test results. She also kept a file of her medical diagnoses, tests, and treatments for future reference.

All women should request copies of their test results and should maintain their own medical records. They should not accept statements like "Your cholesterol level is high." or "Your bone density report is acceptable." from their physician without sufficient documentation.

Natural Transitions in a Woman's Life Are Not Diseases
This principle states that events such as menstruation, menopause, pregnancy, and breast-feeding are normal occurrences in a woman's life and are *not* disease states. Many doctors are taught otherwise, and in my opinion, the American tradition of medical education as a whole is biased against women. I have observed that some male and female physicians provide gender-specific care, but others do not. It is as if medical school and residency training consider the female patient from an antiquated

male viewpoint, and many women accept that perspective as truth.

In medical school and residency training, the concepts of female bodily functions are sometimes described as abnormal states, deviations from the norm, or disease-like conditions. In medical schools, male faculty members and researchers greatly outnumber their female counterparts, and certain events unique to women are often not openly embraced. During my own medical training, the few female faculty members with whom I interacted did not openly discuss their home and family life. Photos of children and spouses were absent from their offices, and their pregnancies were not celebrated. Some women physicians applying for a leadership position in medicine even denied that they had children.

Now I display photos of my husband and children in my office and never hesitate to answer patients' questions about my home and family, but during my residency, I hid my first pregnancy from faculty members and colleagues. I was concerned about their negative responses. To fit in with the male-dominated world of medicine, we women physicians had to deny or downplay our female traits. Our male colleagues seemed to assume that we did not gestate, urinate, menstruate, or lactate.

During my medical training, I once was "scrubbing in" with the chief surgeon before we entered the surgical suite. As I introduced myself, he bellowed at me, "Can you fry meat?" Somewhat confused, I answered affirmatively, that yes, I knew how to cook. He asked, "Can you make babies?" I stated that yes, I assumed that I could bear children, although I had none. He then shouted, " If you can fry meat and make babies, then why the heck do you want to be in my operating room?" I replied, "Well, sir, I believe that women are good for more than just fry-ing meat and making babies," before I stomped into the operating room.

At one point in my training, male and female physicians and medical students shared certain quarters. I recall a loud complaint from a male faculty member, who said that the communal bathroom "smelled like a woman." I then enlisted one of my female colleagues to assist me in transforming that bathroom into a "women's restroom." We hung pantyhose from the shower rod, placed tampons and sanitary napkins on the counters, and positioned bras, hairspray, lipstick, and curling irons in the room. The next day, not one of the male physicians made a single comment, but some of them walked a considerable distance to use a different restroom.

The attitudes pertaining to women physicians in medical school are also applied to female patients and are partly responsible for the lack of optimal care for women. A nurse who held a very senior position at a veterans administration (VA) hospital once described the care provided there for US women veterans in the early 1990s. At the initial high-level meeting about ensuring that VA hospitals provided adequate medical care for female veterans, the first (and presumably most important) item on the agenda stated that women patients would provide their own sanitary napkins. Women were (and still are) one of the most rapidly increasing groups of veterans in this country. They have made great sacrifices in military service. Unfortunately, they have also been victims of gender disparity in medical care, but that trend may be changing. The Center for Women Veterans in Washington, DC, has made tremendous strides in providing gender-specific health care for women who have served in the US military.

Unfortunately, some physicians still expect no questions from their female patients. It is extremely important that all women refuse to be intimidated by such condescension. They *must* demand responsiveness, compassion, and excellence in clinical care from their doctors and access to full information about the status of their health.

Women Are Rational, Social, Emotional, and Spiritual Beings

Nearly 20 years of research in the area of the mind-body connection has revealed that physical and emotional health are inseparably entwined.[22-25] In American medicine, however, the treatment of women is often compartmentalized into two types: either repairing the body without considering the patient's social, psychologic, cultural, and spiritual condition, or erroneously attributing physical symptoms solely to emotional causes. It is very important to select a physician who considers all aspects of a patient's life, in addition to medical history and current physical condition, before a diagnosis is reached and treatment is prescribed. Countless examples from my medical practice and research, like those described below, support that concept.

Reading Between the Lines

One of my patients was a victim of domestic violence. She was being treated with prescription medications for diabetes, high blood pressure, headaches, insomnia, depression, high cholesterol and triglyceride levels, and joint pain. As we developed our patient-physician relationship and established trust, she confided in me and described the abuse she suffered at home. I gave her information about shelters and a crisis hotline, but she doubted that she would have the motivation and courage to leave her husband. She was ashamed because this was her second marriage to an abusive man; she had made the same mistake twice and judged herself harshly for that reason.

I offered emotional support and did not force my opinion, although I advised her of several options and of my desire to help her. Over the following months, she made the decision to leave her marriage. After she did so, her transformation was dramatic and remarkable. She lost 30 pounds (see chapter 6 on how stress contributes to weight gain) and was able to control her diabetes by changing her diet. Her high blood pressure, headaches, joint pain, insomnia, and elevated cholesterol and triglyceride levels either improved or resolved so that no prescription medications were necessary. Her depression lifted as her self-esteem increased. She found a job that she enjoyed, and she established a new social support system for her new life.

The Importance of Being Taken Seriously
Years ago, when I was treating patients in an urgent care facility during a busy holiday season, I was called to examine a woman who complained of headache. The nurse on duty commented to me that this was the woman's fifth visit for headache treatment in a few weeks' time and that "she probably just wanted narcotics." When I greeted the patient, she seemed worried and anxious. She stated that she had recently moved to the area and didn't yet have a personal physician, so she sought help from the urgent care facility when her headaches were severe. She had been Christmas shopping that day and was far from completing her gift buying, decorating, and cooking for her family, but her headache was so intense that she could not continue. She was very concerned about how to fulfill her many social and family obligations when her headache was so debilitating. It was clear to me that she was not seeking narcotics.

I reviewed the patient's chart and noticed that although she had visited the medical facility 4 times, she had never undergone a physical examination. In each case, before being sent home she had received an analgesic injection and a prescription to treat what was presumed to be migraine. I suspected that this patient's headaches were not migraine or stress-related, and I conducted a thorough physical examination that included evaluations of her brain and nervous system. The results of a brain scan revealed that she had 2 brain lesions, which appeared to be malignant. Subsequent tests revealed that the lesions were metastases from a past melanoma. Had this woman's complaint been taken seriously during any of her 4 prior visits, her disease would have been diagnosed and her treatment initiated months earlier.

More and more of my female patients have told me that their health-related complaints are often casually dismissed by doctors who attribute their symptoms to an emotional cause and seldom perform a physical examination.

The Physician Is a Guide, Not a God
Women must refuse to participate in the patriarchal hierarchy of American medical care in which the physician issues orders and commands and the patient listens passively and is shuffled from test to test and specialist to specialist. The physician should serve as a guide who listens to the patient, answers her questions, and works as a partner (sometimes with other specialists) to provide the best treatment. The benefit of a conventional, complementary, or alternative modality should never be dismissed, and the well-being of the patient should be the sole focus of care. Research shows that a physician's humanism (the concern for the patient's dignity and freedom of choice) is a key factor in whether patients follow recommendations about exercise, nutrition, smoking, and maintaining good health.[26]

The Physician Should Be a Role Model of Self-Care

Doctors are often viewed as a role model for proactive health care. In a recent study, 2 groups of physicians counseled their patients about diet and lifestyle.[27] One group consisted of physicians with a normal body weight, and those in the other group were clinically obese. Patients treated by a nonobese physician were significantly more receptive to medical advice about an illness or counseling about wellness practices than were those treated by an obese physician. Another study showed that the relatively healthful diet-related habits of women physicians were related to the likelihood of their counseling patients about nutrition and weight.[28]

Physicians who caution their patients about eating poorly; being addicted to drugs, smoking, or alcohol; not exercising; relying on caffeine and sugar to boost energy; and being a perfectionist or a workaholic should strive to avoid such practices in their own life and work. By doing so, they provide the model of a healthful lifestyle for their patients. I remind my medical students that we cannot expect our patients to be healthier than we ourselves are willing to be or to make lifestyle changes that we would be unwilling to make.

In summary, then, each of us is the guardian of her own health. We must aggressively seek the best in clinical care from physicians who view women as whole, rational, competent people; who do not dismiss symptoms and complaints as being hysterical in nature; and who care for their patients of either gender with intelligence and compassion.

References

1. Rathore SS, Chen J, Wang Y, Radford MJ, Vaccarino V, Krumholz HM. Sex differences in cardiac catheterization: the role of physician gender. *JAMA*. 2001;286(22):2849-2856.

2. Gibler WB, Armstrong PW, Ohman EM, et al. Persistence of delays in presentation and treatment for patients with acute myocardial infarction: The GUSTO-I and GUSTO-III experience. *Ann Emerg Med*. 2002;39(2):123-130.

3. Arnold AL, Milner KA, Vaccarino V. Sex and race differences in electrocardiogram use (the National Hospital Ambulatory Medical Care Survey). *Am J Cardiol*. 2001;88(9):1037-1040.

4. Vakili BA, Kaplan RC, Brown DL. Sex-based differences in early mortality of patients undergoing primary angioplasty for first acute myocardial infarction. *Circulation*. 2001;104(25):3034-3038.

5. Marcuccio E, Loving N, Bennett SK, Hayes SN. A survey of attitudes and experiences of women with heart disease. *Womens Health Issues*. 2003;13(1):23-31.

6. US Department of Health and Human Services. The Office on Women's Health Web site. Available at: www.4woman.gov. Accessed June 16, 2004.

7. Cannon JG, St Pierre BA. Gender differences in host defense mechanisms. *J Psychiatr Res*. 1997;31(1):99-113.

8. Daun JM, Ball RW, Cannon JG. Glucocorticoid sensitivity of interleukin-1 agonist and antagonist secretion: the effects of age and gender. *Am J Physiol Regul Integr Comp Physiol*. 2000;278(4):R855-R862.

9. Rider V, Foster RT, Evans M, Suenaga R, Abdou NI. Gender differences in autoimmune diseases: estrogen increases calcineurin expression in systemic lupus erythematosus. *Clin Immunol Immunopathol*. 1998;89(2):171-180.

10. Whitacre CC, Reingold SC, O'Looney PA. A gender gap in autoimmunity. *Science*. 1999;283(5406):1277-1278.

11. Zang EA, Wynder EL. Differences in lung cancer risk between men and women: examination of the evidence. *J Natl Cancer Inst*. 1996;88(3-4):183-192.

12. Gan TJ, Glass PS, Sigl J, et al. Women emerge from general anesthesia with propofol/alfentanil/nitrous oxide faster than men. *Anesthesiology*. 1999;90(5):1283-1287.

13. Gear RW, Miaskowski C, Gordon NC, Paul SM, Heller PH, Levine JD. The kappa opioid nalbuphine produces gender- and dose-dependent analgesia and antianalgesia in patients with postoperative pain. *Pain*. 1999;83(2):339-345.

14. Mogil JS, Wilson SG, Chesler EJ, et al. The melanocortin-1 receptor gene mediates female-specific mechanisms of analgesia in

mice and humans. *Proc Natl Acad Sci U S A.* 2003;100(8):4867-4872. Epub 2003 Mar 27.

15. Thurmann PA, Hompesch BC. Influence of gender on the pharmacokinetics and pharmacodynamics of drugs. *Int J Clin Pharmacol Ther.* 1998;36(11):586-590.

16. Nishizawa S, Benkelfat C, Young SN, et al Differences between males and females in rates of serotonin synthesis in human brain. *Proc Natl Acad Sci U S A.* 1997;94(10):5308-5313.

17. Rabinowicz T, Dean DE, Petetot JM, de Courten-Myers GM. Gender differences in the human cerebral cortex: more neurons in males; more processes in females. *J Child Neurol.* 1999;14(2):98-107.

18. Department of Health and Human Services. National Institutes of Health. National Heart, Lung, and Blood Institute. Women's Health Initiative. Available at: www.nhlbi.nih.gov/whi. Accessed June 16, 2004.

19. Stephenson K. Hormone replacement therapy. *Panhandle Health.* 1998;18(5):36-38.

20. Hersh AL, Stefanick ML, Stafford RS. National use of postmenopausal hormone therapy: annual trends and response to recent evidence. *JAMA.* 2004;291(1):47-53.

21. Achterberg J. *Woman As Healer.* Boston, Mass: Shambhala Publications; 1991:144-168.

22. Uchino BN, Cacioppo JT, Kiecolt-Glaser JK. The relationship between social support and physiological processes: a review with emphasis on underlying mechanisms and implications for health. *Psychol Bull.* 1996;119(3):488-531.

23. Rein G, Atkinson M, McCraty R The physiological and psychological effects of compassion and anger. *J Adv Med.* 1995;8(2):87-105.

24. McCraty R, Atkinson M, Tiller WA, Rein G, Watkins AD. The effects of emotions on short-term power spectrum analysis of heart rate variability. *Am J Cardiol.* 1995;76(14):1089-1093. Erratum in: *Am J Cardiol.* 1996;77(4):330.

25. Kiecolt-Glaser JK, McGuire L, Robles TF, Glaser R. Psychoneuroimmunology: psychological influences on immune function and health. *J Consult Clin Psychol.* 2002;70(3):537-547.

26. Hauck FR, Zyzanski SJ, Alemagno SA, Medalie JH. Patient perceptions of humanism in physicians: effects on positive health behaviors. *Fam Med.* 1990;22(6):447-452.

27. Hash RB, Munna RK, Vogel RL, Bason JJ. Does physician weight affect perception of health advice? *Prev Med.* 2003;36(1):41-44.

28. Frank E, Wright EH, Serdula MK, Elon LK, Baldwin G. Personal and professional nutrition-related practices of US female physicians. *Am J Clin Nutr.* 2002;75(2):326-332.

Chapter 2
The Feminine Life Cycle

Roma H, whose poetry is featured in this chapter, captures the Golden Mean of Athena (balance in life) in her writing and has embodied it throughout all phases of her life. The mother of 3, she balanced the demands of family life with the challenges of a long career as a successful writer and editor. She has always demonstrated her deep love for her husband and children (and now for her grandchildren, great-grandchildren, and cat, Charlie). She has said that prayer and faith have sustained her during difficult times, and she places great value on her spiritual goals and practice. A loyal friend, she inspires others to live their life with hope and optimism. She volunteers in her church community and regularly visits invalids who depend on others for daily care. Roma is now in her eighth decade of life. Undaunted by the changes of aging, she continues to paint, write, and compose poetry. She has displayed courage during times of great adversity and continues to bless others with her warm nature, creativity, and encouragement.

In contemporary Western social and medical literature, the feminine life cycle is often defined solely by female reproductive status. During my medical training, the term "three bloods" (menarche [the first menstrual period], menstruation, and menopause) was used to refer to the prominent life stages of women. In many aspects of American culture, the most valued feminine attributes are the "three Ms": maidenhood, matrimony, and motherhood.

Only a Pair of Ovaries?

When I was a medical student, I was once a member of a surgical team trying to save the life of a teenage girl who had been shot in the abdomen. She had been dumped from a car onto the sidewalk outside our hospital emergency room around midnight. When she was found, she was unconscious and in shock because of massive blood loss, and several of her internal organs had been severely damaged. The surgery team spent hours in the operating room trying to save her life. Around 5:00 AM, 3 men arrived at the hospital to volunteer the details of the incident.

The patient had shot herself after her boyfriend ended their relationship. Her friends, who were too afraid to call an ambulance, had dumped her on the curb near the hospital. The former boyfriend was one of the 3 men who had come forward with information. The chief resident explained the patient's injuries and her life-threatening condition and asked whether anyone had a question. The ex-boyfriend replied, "Doc, I just have one question: Are her female parts all right?" I was infuriated by that comment. It was clear that in his opinion, the worth of this young woman depended on her ability to function sexually.

That unfortunate view of women is embedded in medical tradition. Emphasis on the value of female reproductive organs and the implication that women are inferior to men is captured in ancient medical doctrines. Aristotle

(384 – 322 BC), for example, stated that the "female state" was a deformity caused by the incomplete development of feminine reproductive organs, which remained inside the body cavity and not in full view, like those of men.[1] Through the influence of the Greek anatomist and physician Claudius Galen (ca 130 – 200), that concept, which persisted through the Middle Ages, was coupled with theologic and philosophic views of women as inferior beings.[2] The theory that the reproductive organs of women rendered them inferior to men remained popular during the Renaissance,[2] and the effects of those teachings are reflected today in Western biomedical attitudes and beliefs.

In 1873 in competition for Harvard University's prestigious Boylston Medical Prize, Mary Putnam Jacobi, MD, submitted her research titled "Do women require mental and bodily rest during menstruation, and to what extent?" Dr. Jacobi had found that, in direct opposition to the popular medical opinions of that time, continuing normal work patterns enabled women to better tolerate menstrual distress. She won the Boylston competition, but when the judges discovered that the winning monograph had been written by a woman, debate about awarding the prize to her ensued.[3]

Nearly a century later, David Reuben, MD, author of *Everything You Always Wanted to Know About Sex But Were Afraid to Ask*, made the following observation about menopausal women: "Having outlived their ovaries, they may have outlived their usefulness as human beings. The remaining years may be just marking time until they follow their glands into oblivion."[4] Those statements reflect American cultural attitudes about menopause in 1970.

Although a women's reproductive status is an important factor in planning her medical care, the view that women are limited by gender alone has always been disturbing to me. It creates the foundation for attitudes and medical practices that have not served women well.

A New Definition of Life's Transitions

According to the value systems described previously, a woman older than 40 years who isn't married or hasn't borne a child becomes devalued and defeminized. But women are more than a walking womb. Many older women are vibrant, influential, productive achievers with rewarding careers and satisfying relationships. A woman's reproductive status (the number of pregnancies and deliveries, the date of the last menstrual period, the choice of contraception) must never solely define her medical care.

A century ago, the average life span of the American woman was 50 years. Today, most nonsmoking American women live to be almost 80 years of age.[5] The average age of menopause (50 years), however, has not changed since the early 1900s.[6] Today, about one third of an American woman's life is lived after menopause, and those decades can be just as rewarding and fulfilling as earlier years. In view of this, I propose a new definition of the feminine life cycle: The three bloods and the three Ms are replaced by love, faith (intuition), and service, which are elements of every woman's life, regardless of socioeconomic status, ethnic heritage, educational level, medical history, stress level, or age (Figure).

The Strength of Love

Love is one of the most powerful emotions. Its absence or presence profoundly influences every human life and has often shifted the course of history. Many women are oriented toward the dream of romantic love; of finding a life partner who will rescue them and transport them, like a princess in a fairy tale, to the realm of "happily ever

Figure. The Feminine Life Cycle

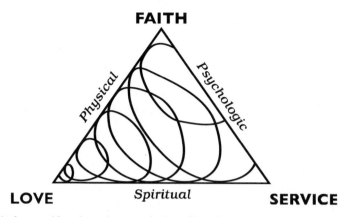

The feminine life cycle revolves around values of love, faith, and service. The first third of the cycle is devoted to physical development; the middle third, to psychologic development; and the final third, to a woman's continued capacity for spiritual growth. The central spiral represents the psyche or soul.

after." Not surprisingly, the emotion of romantic love has a powerful physiologic effect: It evokes a neurochemical response similar to that caused by amphetamines.[7,8] For that reason, our perceptions of life and of other people change when we are romantically in love. The sky seems more blue and the grass, more green. Sensory perception is more acute. Circumstances that previously frustrated or angered us have little effect. Women fueled by romantic love often have more energy and less need for food or sleep. They are primed biologically and culturally to experience romantic love and subsequent mating.

In most women, however, love is not limited to the romantic phase of a relationship but is expressed in various forms throughout life. Since antiquity, women have demonstrated self-love by enhancing their physical attractiveness with cosmetics, perfumes, and fashionable attire. Love for others is also expressed in many ways. Some women are devoted to protecting the environment or caring for animals. Others display love for family, religion, community, or the arts, or they express their love by baking, cooking, or decorating. Many busy mothers take the time to nurture both the body and the spirit by drawing a heart on a sandwich bag as they pack a school lunch.

The Power of Faith and Intuition
Faith is fueled by spiritual beliefs and experiences as well as by intuition, which guides us in making life choices. The strength, steadfastness, and loyalty of women is recounted across centuries and in all cultures. In the Christian tradition, faithful women were described as being last at the cross and first at the grave. According to a Cheyenne proverb, a nation is not conquered until the hearts of its women are on the ground.

The faith of a woman is a powerful force indeed. However, many of my female patients who have expressed a strong spiritual belief often have little confidence in their intuition, which is faith in one's own perceptions (even those that seem illogical or irrational to others). A woman in my care reported that several years ago, she had been diagnosed by another physician as having an estrogen-dependent breast cancer. After she underwent mastectomy, her doctor recommended treatment with tamoxifen, a synthetic drug that blocks various estrogen receptors to prevent cancer recurrence. Tamoxifen therapy, however, may cause the formation of blood clots. As this was explained to the patient, she felt a strange sensation in her chest and had a strong intuitive sense that if she took the drug, she would experience that adverse effect. She rejected treatment with tamoxifen, but her physician pressured her to reconsider. He told her that she had made the wrong decision, that she was not being fair to her husband and children, and that she was indulging in a death wish if she refused treatment. When she remained steadfast, he dismissed her as a patient for refusing to follow his medical advice. She then found another physician, who also strongly recommended treatment with tamoxifen and convinced this woman to take the drug despite her strong inclination to do the opposite. A few weeks after treatment was initiated, she became short of breath and felt a tightness in her chest. Those symptoms became so severe that she sought treatment in a local emergency department, where a pulmonary embolism (a blood clot in the lungs) was diagnosed. This patient later wished that she had followed her intuition and had sought a different effective treatment that did not increase the risk of embolism.

Patients who feel strongly about treatment options should not be intimidated by their physician but should instead have faith in their intuition and search for other effective therapies.

A local newspaper recently featured an account of intuition that saved a life.[9] According to that source, NJ, a retired radio talk show host, began to suffer severe intractable ear pain that did not respond to treatment and eventually became unbearable. A series of local physicians could not determine the cause of the pain. NJ and his wife had been close friends of JB, a young man, also a radio talk show host, who had recently died of a rare hereditary disease. JB collected teddy bears, one of which had been given to NJ and his wife as a memento at the young man's funeral. As her husband suffered, NJ's wife gazed often at the bear. When she walked by it, she thought that she could hear the voice of JB saying, "Call Dad." One night, desperate and unable to relieve her husband's pain, she told him about hearing JB's voice and about her intuition that she should indeed place the call. NJ agreed, but he admonished her not to reveal that she was communicating with teddy bears.

JB's father was a pharmaceutical representative who had connections within the local medical community. He immediately arranged for NJ's examination by a team of physicians, who diagnosed malignant otitis externa, a rare and often fatal infection of the ear and base of the skull. Had that undetected infection progressed much further, cure would not have been possible, but aggressive antibiotic therapy proved successful after a protracted course of treatment. NJ and his wife are certain that her intuition was the key to his recovery. Her action, based only on an inner knowing, made the difference between his life and death.

The Rewards of Service

A concerned group of women united by service can make the impossible possible. Service is a form of nurturing others, helping the community, and furthering causes. Many women sacrifice their own needs to answer the demands of work, friends, and family. They organize, plan, and execute social events such as bridal showers, weddings, graduations, baby showers, and funerals. Almost all my women patients have at some time volunteered to assist a worthy cause. Their community service takes various forms: preparing food for bake sales, organizing and participating in fundraisers, leading a prayer circle or book study group, caring for abandoned animals, or visiting patients in nursing homes, older people, and those with a disability. I often prescribe such involvement for my women patients who have never volunteered for a special cause. Service to others provides a host of emotional and spiritual benefits for those who perform it.

When Love, Faith, Intuition, and Service Are Missing

When life is out of balance, the antitheses of love, faith, intuition, and service develop in work and intimate relationships. I frequently ask my female patients if they are most often motivated by guilt, fear, and obligation. If so, that toxic combination over time adversely affects physical and emotional health (see the appendices). If motivation for the wrong reasons becomes the norm, it is important to seek help from a physician, a spiritual or religious leader, or a counselor to restore perspective and develop effective coping skills.

Phases of the Feminine Life Cycle

For many American women, the feminine life cycle encompasses almost 90 years. Each season of life brings its own rewards and challenges, but throughout them all, the emotional, social, cultural, and spiritual aspects of living are as important as physical health to our well-being. Those attributes change at 3 age plateaus in the feminine life cycle. Physical development is paramount from infancy to 30 years of age; psychologic growth, from 30 to 60 years; and spiritual development at roughly 60 years or older. Women may find health of the body, mind, and spirit elusive when they resist progressing to the next phase of development or if their progress to the next phase is too rapid.

Phase I: Physical Development

During the first third of a woman's life (birth to 30 years), her physical development is amazing. As an infant, her physical coordination develops rapidly as she becomes more interactive with her environment. As a child, she acquires verbal fluency with ease and acquires the ability for abstract reasoning. At the midpoint in the first phase of the feminine life cycle (about the age of 12 years), she experiences puberty. Reproductive organs develop, and menstruation occurs. At this stage of life, a young woman's muscles are flexible, and her bones are strong. Her senses are acute, and her cardiovascular and immune systems are robust as they continue to develop. Her intellect is sharp, and she quickly learns and processes new information. In late adolescence, most American women become independent from the family unit and secure a job, a car, and an apartment. In that phase of life, hormonal changes create an instinctual and powerful interest in coupling that competes with compelling professional and social interests.

Phase II: Psychologic Growth
In the second third of the feminine life cycle (30 to 60 years), psychologic growth and development are emphasized. By the age of 30 years, the typical American woman has selected a career and defined a life path. She may have chosen marriage and motherhood, or her career may be her sole focus. Greater demands on her time and energy may cause her to abandon some activities of self-nurture, such as regular exercise. Her body may have changed dramatically as a result of pregnancy, illness, or injury.

As she is challenged by interactions with others at work and with family at home, a woman in the second phase of life begins to mature emotionally and psychologically. She learns that statements like "You have a noble and lofty vision." really mean that the boss thinks she can't achieve her goal. She begins to understand the meaning of the "good old boy" network and begins negotiating and compromising to meet her goals. She learns about the give-and-take of the adult world and becomes emotionally mature. Sublimation, altruism, and humor become useful in managing conflicts. She becomes adept at multitasking while carrying on an active inner life. She is immersed in the practical world. On an average weekday morning before going to work, a "30-something" mother might comfort her preschooler, prepare lunches for her school-age children, address a birthday card to her sister-in-law, finish a load of laundry, remind her husband about a PTA meeting, prepare the evening meal in a Crock-Pot, feed her children breakfast, give the dog its medicine, and counsel her second-grader about how to respond to a conflict at school. This woman has learned to expect the unexpected; perhaps a call for help from a co-worker who was up most of the night with a sick child and is now late for work. She might agree to cover for her friend as her children wait for her in the car, and her work day begins.

Problems often arise when women in this phase of life ignore their own emotional needs in their quest to be a perfect mother. One of my patients in her early 30s began to experience dizziness, episodes in which she nearly fainted, and chest pain. Her physical examination and medical tests revealed a minor heart problem, but her symptoms were so severe that she was hospitalized during the Christmas holidays. This patient, a leader in her community, had 4 children younger than 10 years of age, and she home-schooled her older children. She was intensely focused on the well-being of her family and on her own spiritual journey of motherhood, parenting, nurturing, and teaching her children. She was careful to always set a perfect example for her children in her speech, behavior, meal preparation, lesson plans, and household duties. She stated that she had never been separated from her 2 toddlers for more than a few hours because she was still nursing them, which had become a spiritual experience for her.

During her office visits and social interactions, this patient expressed none of the frustrations and complaints (sleepless nights, an endless number of dirty diapers, a lack of privacy) that typically pepper the conversations of young mothers. I believe that her physical symptoms stemmed in part from her strong emphasis on her spiritual role as a mother and the neglect of her self-concept as a wife and individual. Over time, the denial of her own emotional needs and the repression of conflicts contributed to her physical decline and emotional atrophy.

In the latter part of the second phase of life (about the age of 45 years), a midlife transition occurs. Many women then begin to seek authenticity in their work and search for relationships that balance inner values with external reality. They begin to realize their own mortality and may reflect on lost dreams and missed opportunities. As their children mature and leave home or family obligations diminish, many of these women find freedom, develop creative insight, and identify new outlets for self-development. Others may assume the demanding role of caregiver for an ill spouse or parent.

Phase III: Spiritual Development
The final phase of the feminine life cycle involves spiritual growth and development. Women in this stage of life are not afraid to speak the truth loudly and clearly. They no longer feel the need to hide their feelings, and they prefer honesty to convention. Women older than 60 years face retirement, widowhood, cross-country moves, and income reduction. A healthy response to those transitions brings new friendships, activities, interests, and hobbies. I had the honor of meeting Syntha West, PhD, who was voted Ms. Senior Texas several years ago. Dr. West enjoyed a successful career as a psychologist. When she retired in her 60s, she embarked on reclaiming a lost dream: to compete in a beauty pageant. She took lessons in singing, dancing, and piano and achieved more than her goal; she won the competition.

One of my patients also realized a lifelong dream during her senior years. Despite chronic health problems, she and her beloved border collie entered their first competition in dog agility. She eventually created a dog agility course in her backyard and began to offer training in that sport, which brought together a diverse group of dog owners with a common interest. Her endeavors brought pleasure and purpose to many people, including my family. At her invitation, my daughters and I attended our first dog agility trials, which we enjoyed tremendously.

In the third phase of the feminine life cycle, emphasizing physical attributes rather than spiritual strengths can be a source of problems. One of my patients, a college-educated widow in her 70s, lived near her daughter and grandchildren. During her first visit to my office, she commented on the appearance of her hands and then asked me about possible prescription treatments to eliminate brown liver spots, a common skin condition and natural sign of aging. I discussed treatment options with her in addition to providing other healthcare advice. During each subsequent appointment, she expressed discontent about various natural signs of growing older, but she was most often dissatisfied about the appearance of her hands. She compared them unfavorably with my hands, the nurse's hands, and those of others with whom she interacted. I once gently suggested that she might consider wearing lace gloves if the sight of her hands was so unsettling, but she strongly rejected that idea.

Eventually, this patient experienced a medical urgency, and I was the physician on call. I was amazed that even in the urgent care department, she continued to comment on the appearance of her hands and how ugly they were. As I examined her, she demanded to see my hands and commented on my good fortune because I had no liver spots. The appearance of her hands remained inordinately important to her. She did not experience pleasure from her good health or the company of her grandchildren but was consumed instead with negativism about the natural process of aging.

Advancing age is accompanied by decreasing independence or even institutionalization, and some women in the third phase of life focus on loss, loneliness, and other problems of aging. They become socially and emotionally isolated, and their life eventually becomes the dreary prospect that they fear most. A positive outlook helps accomplish even the most difficult transitions with dignity and grace. Age-related physical changes (reduced vision and hearing, progressive osteoarthritis, diminished physical endurance) can be minimized by a spirit that remains alive and vibrant.

> Appendices B and C in this book list activities designed for older women with health limitations. I have found that with guidance, support, and the belief that serenity can be achieved, negative attitudes change for the better and the quality of life improves.

One of my patients oversees medical care for her mother, JD, who is institutionalized because of severe Alzheimer's disease. A young female caregiver at the residential care facility commented that JD was a great inspiration. That statement was confusing to my patient, because her mother had no short-term memory and could not function independently as the vibrant, intelligent, active woman she had been before her illness. The compliment made perfect sense to me, though. JD's spirit, unhampered by intellectual limitations and shaped by decades of a generous and caring life, remained the most enduring element of her personality.

The Central Spiral
Throughout all phases of the feminine life cycle, a complex force referred to as the "central spiral" remains an

essential element. The central spiral is unique to each woman. It is the essence of the individual feminine psyche; the soulful, innermost part of the female self that is moved by a touch, a song, or a painting. It is the inner source of immense joy or wrenching pain that differs for each of us. It is the core of the will to live. The central spiral is not a rational force and has no linear progression; it is fluid and ever-changing in response to attitude, experience, and perception. It powerfully links past experiences with present everyday life. I often keep the concept of each patient's central spiral in mind as I search for a medical diagnosis. If one of my women patients has unexplained physical symptoms, I inquire about anniversary dates of influential events, even decades before, that have shaped the central spiral and the patient's core beliefs.

It is important to remember that as American women, we have many choices in all phases of life. The voice of Athena, the advocate for balance in living, resonates within us all. Listening to that intuition enables us — at any age — to make the choices that best serve us and those we love.

References

1. *Aristotle. On the Generation of Animals.*

2. Walton MT, Fineman RM, Walton PJ. Why can't a woman be more like a man? A renaissance perspective on the biological basis for female inferiority. *Women Health.* 1996;24(4):87-95.

3. Achterberg AJ. *Woman as Healer.* Boston, Mass: Shambhala Publications; 1991:150-152.

4. Reuben DR. *Everything You Always Wanted to Know About Sex But Were Afraid to Ask.* New York, NY: Bantam Books, Inc; 1970:366.

5. Arias E. United States life tables, 2001. *National Vital Statistics Reports.* 2004;52(14). Available at: www.cdc.gov/nchs/data/nvsr/nvsr52/nvsr52_14.pdf. Accessed June 22, 2004.

6. Berg G, Hammar M. *The Modern Management of the Menopause.* Pearl River, NY: Parthenon Publishing Group; 1994:17-23.

7. Ackerman D. *A Natural History of Love.* New York, NY: Vintage Books; 1995.

8. Liebowitz MR. *The Chemistry of Love.* Boston, Mass: Little, Brown & Company; 1984.

9. Taravella E. Johnson using faith to fight disease. *The Daily Sentinel.* June 5, 2004:1.

Author's Note: *I have had the privilege of serving as a physician for thousands of women in their 60s, 70s, 80s, and older. Many of those patients have responded to illness, physical challenge, and personal loss with strength, compassion, and grace that has been more than inspiring. Safeguarding the health of some of these patients is so uplifting that I eagerly await their appointments; just seeing their names on the schedule is encouraging. One such patient is Roma H, to whom this chapter is dedicated. She has graciously allowed me to include her poems at the close of this chapter.*

Although Roma is now in her late 70s and struggles with several chronic illnesses, she exhibits a youthful enthusiasm that is energizing. She can remember and appreciate her youth, but she also enjoys the present and looks forward to the future. Her poems, which capture the essence of her life view, appear below.

When I Was Young
Roma H

When I was young, life was easy living amid the blossoming fruit. I did child things, thought child thoughts as I walked barefoot on the green.

Life was free and simple as a singing brook flowing in facile beauty. And oft' my friend, the new, young sun took me through the day — from dawn's first thin gleam upon red berries ready to pluck, then on to the intense gold rebuke of high noon as morn's lively leaves nodded into a brief siesta.

Too soon Old Sol colored the evening, shooting his rays on vermilion cliffs to the west and transforming the dull, black lava of the east into shining ebony.

Over and over the sun was reborn — as the Phoenix from its gray ash — giving his life, his warmth and light to every living thing — yet at times burning harsh, angry darts of fire in a relentless, immovable brilliant blaze.

Then, seeking refuge 'neath the protective green limbs of my favorite walnut tree — I could read a tale, dream a dream, write a poem, sing a song, or wish to be a lovely, shining princess of rare beauty, or perhaps a friend would join me and we'd giggle about whimsical things.

There were afternoons of lying in the grass watching clouds paint their nebulous pictures. Happy days, doing chores, tasting fresh, juicy ripe fruit — peaches, apricots, plums, pomegranates, cherries....

Many an eve I remember sitting in the back yard round a campfire with family — almost grasping a thread — a hint of primal memory as I savored food made hot 'neath the glowing coals.

Most summers I remember going with family to Cedar Mountain and sleeping under the sky, its midnight-blue illumined by other worlds of light, and wondering if someone in that supernal splendor was breathing in awe o'er the light of planet earth.

And suddenly the red-orange-gold of autumn loomed. A new tingle pricked my being with thoughts of pre-life friends, real or imagined. And I'd wonder what it was like before I joined my earth family.

Then it seemed that in almost a blink of an eye, autumn came to let summer rest. Soon I was fed with learning with the stale familiarity of busy school days, of freedom — days of growing seemed to disappear as quickly as new-churned butter on a hot ear of homegrown corn. And in its place came a different kind of learning — a time of absorption — a time of balance — a new agenda — a new map.

Form. Steel. Glass. Concrete. Challenge. Winning — being the best that I can be.

Child Roma
Roma H

She was ever walking on a rail —
Sometimes with pickets close at hand.
She balanced, wobbled — and sometimes fell
On hard earth — not soft grains of sand.
Or she hung from her knees upon a limb —
From her very special walnut tree.
It was her private outside gym —
She would cast a smile in secret glee.
Or she sat and read among the green,
With walnuts ripening on the tree.
Her heart beat with love — and her being
Reached up in thanks — dear Lord to Thee.

Chapter 3
The Golden Mean of Athena:
Living a Balanced Live

This chapter is dedicated to the working women who participated in my clinical research project "Yoga for Working Women" and to yoga expert Lilias Folan. The women in my research project awakened their Athena archetype by becoming aware of the effects of stress on their body and mind and by using the practice of yoga to achieve balance and manage challenges. Lilias Folan, a pioneer in American yoga, has illuminated the path to the Golden Mean for many women through her teaching and her professional and personal dedication to living a balanced life.

Women fulfill multiple roles in American society today, and for many of us, achieving the Golden Mean of Athena, or balance in life, is a challenge. According to a recent survey by the National Women's Health Resource Center, 93% of women respondents reported a moderate-to-high daily stress level.[1] Other research[2,3] has shown that 85% of working women (a term that, in this book, refers to women who work outside the home) felt guilty about combining the demands of work with those of their family. "When I'm working, I think about what I need to do at home, and when I'm at home, I think about what I need to be doing at work," said one of my women patients, and many others have expressed a similar conflict. Women living a modern lifestyle are constantly bombarded with information and demands. Many of us must respond and react to e-mail, voice mail, cellular phones, pagers, electronic media, responsibilities at work, and the demands of a "24-7" lifestyle in addition to the traditional needs of family and community. I have observed repeatedly in my clinical practice that women do not allow themselves adequate time for rest, reflection, and rejuvenation of mind, body, and spirit.

This chapter has a dual purpose: to examine one of the greatest problems faced by contemporary working women (the "double-day" life) and to offer an effective, inexpensive method (the practice of yoga) for restoring a balanced lifestyle. A list of resources at the chapter conclusion offers options for those interested in the benefits of that ancient art.

Stress and Burnout

The conflict between the demands of work and responsibilities at home contributes to burnout, which is the physical and emotional exhaustion caused by prolonged stress. The physical symptoms of burnout include extreme tiredness, headaches, disturbed sleep, and non-specific pain. Among the cognitive and emotional symptoms are loss of idealism and motivation, reduced attention span, feelings of meaninglessness or apathy, and detachment.[4-7] Many working women in my care have experienced burnout, which is common among those in caregiving professions such as nursing, teaching, or social services.

It is not surprising that in 2002, more than 76% of the lost productive time at work in the United States was attributed to stress-related disorders (headaches, back pain, other types of musculoskeletal pain) that are often preventable.[8] Recent data show that reduced perform-ance during work costs an estimated $61.2 billion annu-ally in the United States.[8]

The Double-Day Life

Of the 62 million US women employed in 1999, 46 mil-lion (75%) worked full-time, 16 million (25%) worked part-time, and 3.7 million (approximately 6%) held mul-tiple jobs.[9] Many of those women worked a "double day": eight or more hours at work plus time spent caring for children, spouses, and parents and performing other tasks at home. Since 1999, that stress has not dimin-ished. Working women, who now account for 46% of the 137 million US workers,[10] still defer their own needs to answer those of others. They routinely forgo the self-care that leads to better functioning on all personal and pro-fessional levels.

The Stress of Change

In America today, many job markets are in flux. Recent downsizing in the healthcare industry and other venues has led to a greater workload for individual employees, an increase in the number of rotating shifts assigned to each worker, and an associated increase in work and family conflicts, all of which affect well-being.

Stress levels are often job specific. In 2000, 94.6% of reg-istered nurses in the United States were women.[11] Female nurses reported the greatest degree of job-related strain: Their work is emotionally demanding, imposes extensive responsibility, and provides little control.[2,6] Other studies show that women who most often experience job-related burnout also have a high work-related stress level.[4,5,7]

Failing to "Measure Up"

Stressors other than job-related demands and family needs also affect working women. According to contemporary American culture, happiness for women is a function of being thin; having a happy husband, well-adjusted children, and a successful career; and maintaining a clean and orderly home. Those standards are constantly reinforced in electronic and print media. Achieving them, however, is not possible or practical for many women. Falling short of those standards, they gradually become overwhelmed by self-judgment, guilt, anxiety, and stress. Such negativity adversely affects their health.

"Learned helplessness" often develops when women feel unable to change their circumstances at work or at home, and they give up on themselves and on life.

The Effects of Stress and Anger

Men and women may differ in the types of stress to which they respond most strongly in the workplace. As a family physician, I have observed that working men are most negatively affected by budget issues, the hassle of schedule changes, and technical problems such as computer failure. Working women are most stressed by interpersonal conflict.

Physiologic Effects of Stress

Like the triggers for stress, the physiologic effects of stress may also be gender specific. In women, the cardiovascular response to psychologic stress tends to cause an immediate increase in heart rate and an increased volume of cardiac output, but psychologically stressed men experience an immediate increase in blood pressure and a decrease in blood vessel size.[12-14] Studies show that women under psychologic stress release higher levels of catecholamines (especially adrenaline) than do men under similar stress. Women also experience a prolonged increase in or an abnormally elevated level of cortisol after a psychologically stressful event, but men similarly stressed exhibit a more rapid return of cortisol to the normal baseline level.[12,15-22]

In a research study of the physiologic response to psychologic stress in married couples, the wives (but not the husbands) displayed a significant increase in the levels of catecholamines and cortisol during an emotional conflict.[23] Other research has shown that conflict and chronic stress more often affect immune system function in women than in men.[23-25] Studies indicate that women in caregiver roles are more profoundly affected by the stress-related reduction in endogenous substances that fight infection, inflammation, and tumor development than are women without those responsibilities.[23,25-28]

Emotional conflict causes greater and more persistent physiologic changes in women as opposed to men for several reasons: the effects of the interplay between female reproductive hormones and stress hormones, the greater sensitivity of women to emotional conflict, and a greater incidence in women of frequently intrusive thoughts about stressful experiences over time.[29,26,30-33] Because even memories of stressful events can evoke physiologic changes, the tendency of women to retain more detailed and vivid memories of conflicts may be a disadvantage.[30,34]

Most working women report that their stress level is high, and they also experience more stress-related disorders than do working men.[35] Musculoskeletal disorders (chronic back pain, carpal tunnel syndrome), which represent more than 60% of occupational illnesses, are more common in working women than in men who work.[10] Psychologic stress can cause fatigue, obesity, depression, and certain physical complaints, all of which are common reasons for absenteeism in the female American workforce.[35]

I believe that anger also contributes significantly to illness, especially cardiovascular disease in women. When anger and hostility are repressed over time, feelings of shame, depression, and guilt accumulate and intensify. Repressed anger causes physiologic stress that adversely affects the cardiovascular system (which may increase the risk of heart attack) and also compromises immune system function.[31-33,36,37]

Emotional Effects of Stress

Research indicates that the stress-related response of women subjected to personal harassment differs from their reaction when they defend a friend who is being harassed. In a Canadian study of the physiologic and psychologic effects of interpersonal conflict, 42 women were paired with a close female friend in one of two scenarios.[37] In the "Self-Harass" scenario, the subjects were harassed while performing a math task. In the "Friend-Harass" scenario, the subjects defended their friend, who was harassed while performing a math task. The Self-Harass women experienced significantly greater depression, feelings of guilt, and increases in heart rate, cardiac output, blood pressure, and other cardiovascular responses when they themselves were provoked than when they acted to protect a friend who was being harassed. This implies that the selective response to stress has great potential to affect our overall health.

Yoga: An Ancient Answer to Modern Stress

As I became more aware of the effects of stress, anger, and burnout on my patients and on myself, I began to search for a positive method for creating emotional hardiness, resilience, and the ability to cope. I wanted to find an antidote to the emotional and physical toll taken by the stressful events that we all face in various forms.

In 1996, I found an effective solution. I was introduced to yoga by an incredibly warm and understanding teacher. She was patient and not pushy. Through her direction, I learned to use yoga to relax and rejuvenate in just 60 min-

> Why not organize a yoga class at your workplace? Yoga videos and mats are inexpensive, readily available tools for managing work-related stress. Seated yoga (available on video) can be practiced at your desk.

utes, despite a demanding personal and professional schedule. I discovered that practicing yoga contributes profoundly to maintaining good physical and emotional health.

Physiologic Benefits of Yoga
Yoga is an effective complement to traditional medical care and an alternative to drug therapy for many disorders, including depression, anxiety, obsessive-compulsive behavior, premenstrual syndrome, and the symptoms of menopause or aging. Yoga also improves physical function by increasing flexibility and strengthening muscles, and it increases the heart's ability to use oxygen.[38-40] Practicing yoga regularly causes a subsequent prolonged reduction in heart rate and blood pressure, reduces the incidence of stress-related headaches and musculoskeletal pain, inhibits the release of cortisol, and minimizes sympathetic nervous system hyperreactivity in response to stress.[41-47]

Yoga benefits the elderly in many ways. Hyperkyphosis (dowager's hump) is an abnormal curvature of the upper spine caused by aging, osteoporosis, or a compression fracture of a vertebra. In one study, women with hyperkyphosis who ranged in age from 63 to 86 years (average age, 75 years) attended a 1-hour hatha yoga class twice weekly.[48] After 12 weeks, these women exhibited a measurable increase in height and a decrease in forward curvature of the spine, as well as an improvement in physical performance and well-being. This study is exciting to me because it suggests that many elderly women can improve their posture, physical strength, and flexibility simply by adding the practice of yoga to their lifestyle.

Psychologic Benefits of Yoga

Practicing yoga relieves depression and anxiety. Yoga expert Amy Weintraub published a brilliant article on the positive effects of regular practice on depression and anxiety in women.[49] Research indicates that yoga also effectively relieves emotional stress in children,[50] and my daughters and I agree. We have found the deck of cards titled *Kids'Yoga Deck: 50 Poses and Games* (San Francisco, Calif: Books, 2003) especially useful for practicing yoga together at home and when we travel.

The Benefits of Yoga for Women of All Ages

- Increases strength and endurance
- Improves posture and flexibility
- Benefits the cardiovascular system by lowering blood pressure and heart rate and increasing the ability of the heart to use oxygen
- Relieves tension, anxiety, and stress through breathing techniques and controlled movement
- Restores vitality, improves mood, and decreases physical pain
- Enables relaxation, which rejuvenates and restores the mind and the body
- Is inexpensive and can be easily integrated into daily life at work, at home, or even in a hospital bed or wheelchair

---

Stories from the Heart

Over the years, I have recommended the practice of yoga to thousands of women who have reported a successful outcome. One patient shared the following comment:

> When I decided to obtain my college degree, the academic stress was overwhelming. I would lose my temper at the slightest provocation, and my mind would constantly race from one topic to another. It was extremely difficult for me to relax. My family and I were confused by my unusual irritability and lack of concentration. In addition, my face began to break out, and I became depressed. Doctor Stephenson recommended yoga to help reduce stress, balance my hormone levels, and lower my abnormally high cortisol level. Skeptical but desperate, I attended my first yoga class. Afterwards, I felt a sense of peace that returned each time I practiced my yoga postures. I now practice yoga daily, and I continue to experience the same benefits that I noticed after my first session.

> Yoga has taught me to be aware of my body and my breathing. When I feel myself becoming tense, I consciously focus on my breathing and relax my muscles. Those techniques allow me to think and act clearly. Yoga has improved my relationship with friends, family, and God. Before I began to practice regularly, I was so anxious that I could not enjoy anything, but yoga has given me the tools to relax and enjoy life. I am comforted by knowing that I can turn to yoga to relax my mind and body, which gives me a positive outlook on life.

New Research

Investigators from the National Institutes of Health (NIH) are examining the effects of yoga in patients with insomnia, multiple sclerosis, or shortness of breath from chronic obstructive pulmonary disease, as well as the role of yoga in delaying the aging of the human brain.[51] Yoga has many other applications as well. In 2002, when I was working in a state-sponsored university hospital in Texas, I became concerned about the level of stress in our female employees. While at work, they had easy access to caffeine, nicotine, and sugar. I felt that practicing yoga would be a much more healthful alternative to relieving stress on the body, mind, and spirit. To test my opinion, I served as the principal investigator for a research project on the efficacy of yoga in reducing stress in working women.[52]

In that study, a questionnaire that measured quality of life as determined by physical, emotional, and social health was used to evaluate each subject before and after 3 months of once-weekly 60-minute yoga classes. As my staff and I began preparing for the research project, I was told that yoga was "not a Texas thing," that "no one would be interested," and that "women are too stressed out to participate." The room eventually designated for the yoga classes accommodated only 8 to 15 women.

I was not daunted by that skepticism, and we proceeded according to plan. We decided to recruit female employees and volunteers from the hospital health center in which I had my medical practice. Our minimal advertising generated an excellent response: In just a few days, 129 women registered to participate. Eighty-five of the women who applied met the inclusion criteria. We did not include women with uncontrolled high blood pressure or previously undiagnosed problems with the heart, brain, or nervous system.

During the research sessions, hatha yoga (a style that incorporates a combination of breathing and movement) was taught. The program consisted of 12 weeks of video yoga instruction that was offered in one 60-minute session each week. I selected a video series for beginning students (*Lilias' Yoga Workout Series for Beginners* and *Flowing Postures of Yoga*) by Lilias Folan, a certified teacher of hatha yoga, as instruction. Ms. Folan launched the groundbreaking yoga series *Lilias! Yoga and You*, which was featured for 20 years on public broadcasting television stations and was watched by an audience of millions. Her teaching style is warm, encouraging, and dynamic. She is a wife, a mother, a grandmother, and a working woman, as were most of the participants in my research study.

Many of the women in the class had experienced the challenges of a recent or chronic illness and were not able to rise from a seated position on the floor without support. At the end of the 12-week research study, however, all of the participants could rise from the floor without using a prop (an achievement that was very meaningful). No work-related injuries or illnesses were reported during the study. At the end of the project, each participant indicated a significant improvement in all categories of a quality-of-life questionnaire. All the women were better able to perform everyday activities (lifting or carrying groceries, climbing stairs, bending, kneeling, stooping, walking one or more blocks, pushing a vacuum cleaner). They also reported a greater feeling of accomplishment in work and other activites (including household duties), a heightened enjoyment of social activities, a decrease in physical pain, and a sense of feeling less focused on physical and emotional problems. Many noted an overall improvement in their mood and vitality that they described as feeling "less worn out," "more full of life," "less tired," "less nervous," "less down in the dumps," or "having more energy." The results of the study showed that weekly hatha yoga sessions can produce benefits in overall health and are safe and acceptable for most working women. After the study ended, many of the participants continued to practice yoga regularly.

"Bedtop" Yoga: Gentle Practice for Special Cases
For patients who cannot assume hatha yoga poses because of a musculoskeletal or cardiac condition, obesity, or a disability, I recommend Kripalu yoga, which includes "seated" yoga and bedtop yoga. Kripalu yoga is beautifully taught in videos by certified yoga instructor Carol Dickman, who

guides her students through a series of effective but modified poses that can be adapted as necessary. No props are used. Seated yoga is energizing, and bedtop yoga, which is performed from a supine position, promotes tranquility and relaxation. Many of my patients have benefitted from these gentle yoga practices, and some have even gained enough strength and stamina to progress (with their physician's approval) to regular yoga poses.

Recommended Resources for Yoga Practice

Buckley A. *Kids' Yoga Deck: 50 Poses and Games.* San Francisco, Calif: Chronicle Books; 2003 — Annie Buckley is a yoga instructor who created an excellent yoga program for children (kindergarten through fifth grade) at the Los Angeles Accelerated School.

Miller OH, Kaufman N. *The Yoga Deck: 50 Poses & Meditations for Body, Mind & Spirit.* San Francisco, Calif: Chronicle Books, 2001

Scaravelli V. *Awakening the Spine: The Stress-Free Yoga That Works With the Body to Restore Health, Vitality and Energy.* Second edition. San Francisco, Calif: HarperSanFrancisco; 1991 — Especially inspiring for women over 50

Folan L. *Complete Lilias! Yoga Fitness for Beginners (Arms & Abs, Legs, & Buns, Cardio Challenge)* (2000) (DVD; Goldhil Home Media I; 2004) and *Lilias! Am & Pm Yoga Workouts-Seniors* (DVD, Goldhil Home Media I; 2003) — Two excellent yoga videos, audio CDs, cassettes, and DVDs by yoga expert Lilias Folan. Students at any level of proficiency can find instruction from the many programs offered in the series. Available at: www.liliasyoga.com/. Accessed May 19, 2004.

Dickman C. www.stretch.com — Yoga for special circumstances:
Bed Top Yoga. (video) Studio name not available; 1999.
Bed Top Yoga. 1st edition (audio cassette). Yoga Enterprises; 1997.
Seated Yoga. (video) Studio name not available; 1999.
In-Flight Yoga. 1st edition. (audio cassette) Yoga Enterprises; 1997.

[No author listed.] *Yoga at Your Desk* (video; VN Industries, Inc; 2001) Available at: www.yogaatyourdesk.com. — An excellent stress reliever to use at work.

Yoga instruction — Batsheva Steinbeck, PO Box 65561, Tucson, AZ; telephone: 520-529-9120.

Acknowledgement

The author would like to acknowledge the following contributors to the yoga research study of which she was the principal investigator: Barbara Pinson, MD; David

Holiday, PhD; Ron Dodson, PhD; Kathy Hayden, LVN; Patti Harvey; Susan Brown; Judy Robinson; Ellen Remenchek, MD; Amanda Bunt; Anne Perryman; Linda Ahrens; Jeff Levine, MD; and Kevin Roper.

References

1. National Women's Health Resource Center. National Women's Health Report: Women, Chronic Stress and Resilience/June 2003. Available at: www.healthywomen.org/content.cfm?L1=2&CID=93&Blist=19. Accessed June 1, 2004.

2. National Institute for Occupational Safety and Health (NIOSH). *Stress at Work.* Atlanta, Ga: National Institute for Occupational Safety and Health (NIOSH); 1999. Publication No. 99-101. Available at: www.cdc.gov/niosh/atwork.html. Accessed: April 15, 2004.

3. Spurlock J. How stress affects the body. In: *The Women's Complete Healthbook.* Alexandria, Va: The American Medical Women's Association. Available at: www.amwadoc.org/publications/WCHealthbook/stressamwach09.html. Accessed May 16, 2004.

4. Pruessner JC, Hellhammer DH, Kirschbaum C. Burnout, perceived stress, and cortisol responses to awakening. *Psychosom Med.* 1999;61(2):197-204.

5. Beer J, Beer J. Burnout and stress, depression and self-esteem of teachers. *Psychol Rep.* 1992;71(3 Pt 2):1331-1336.

6. Costantini A, Solano L, Di Napoli R, Bosco A. Relationship between hardiness and risk of burnout in a sample of 92 nurses working in oncology and AIDS wards. *Psychother Psychosom.* 1997;66(2):78-82.

7. Maslach C, Schaufeli WB, Leiter MP. Job burnout. *Annu Rev Psychol.* 2001;52:397-422.

8. Stewart WF, Ricci JA, Chee E, Morganstein D, Lipton R. Lost productive time and cost due to common pain conditions in the US workforce. *JAMA.* 2003;290(18):2443-2454.

9. National Institute for Occupational Safety and Health (NIOSH). *Women's Safety and Health Issues at Work.* Available at: www.cdc.gov/niosh/topics/women/. Accessed: June 1, 2004.

10. Messing K. Women's occupational health: a critical review and discussion of current issues. *Women Health.* 1997;25(4):39-68.

11. Spratley E, Johnson A, Sochalski J, Fritz M, Spencer W. *The Registered Nurse Population. March 2000: Findings From the National Sample Survey of Registered Nurses.* Available at:

bhpr.hrsa.gov/healthworkforce/reports/rnsurvey/rnss1.htm. Accessed June 21, 2004.

12. Stoney CM, Matthews KA, McDonald RH, Johnson CA. Sex differences in lipid, lipoprotein, cardiovascular, and neuroendocrine responses to acute stress. *Psychophysiology.* 1988;25(6):645-656.

13. Allen MT, Stoney CM, Owens JF, Matthews KA. Hemodynamic adjustments to laboratory stress: the influence of gender and personality. *Psychosom Med.* 1993;55(6):505-517.

14. Girdler SS, Turner JR, Sherwood A, Light KC. Gender differences in blood pressure control during a variety of behavioral stressors. *Psychosom Med.* 1990;52(5):571-591.

15. Jacobson NS, Gottman JM, Waltz J, Rushe R, Babcock J, Holtzworth-Munroe A. Affect, verbal content, and psychophysiology in the arguments of couples with a violent husband. *J Consult Clin Psychol.* 1994;62(5):982-988.

16. Lundberg U, Frankenhaeuser M. Stress and workload of men and women in high-ranking positions. *Occup Health Psychol.* 1999;4(2):142-151.

17. Brisson C, Laflamme N, Moisan J, Milot A, Masse B, Vezina M. Effect of family responsibilities and job strain on ambulatory blood pressure among white-collar women. *Psychosom Med.* 1999;61(2):205-213.

18. Steptoe A, Lundwall K, Cropley M. Gender, family structure and cardiovascular activity during the working day and evening. *Soc Sci Med.* 2000;50(4):531-539.

19. Luecken LJ, Suarez EC, Kuhn CM, et al. Stress in employed women: impact of marital status and children at home on neurohormone output and home strain. *Psychosom Med.* 1997;59(4):352-359.

20. Kirschbaum C, Wust S, Hellhammer D. Consistent sex differences in cortisol responses to psychological stress. *Psychosom Med.* 1992;54(6):648-657.

21. Adam EK, Gunnar MR. Relationship functioning and home and work demands predict individual differences in diurnal cortisol patterns in women. *Psychoneuroendocrinology.* 2001;26(2):189-208.

22. Sluiter JK, Frings-Dresen MH, Meijman TF, van der Beek AJ. Reactivity and recovery from different types of work measured by catecholamines and cortisol: a systematic literature overview. *Occup Environ Med.* 2000;57(5):298-315.

23. Kiecolt-Glaser JK, Glaser R, Cacioppo JT, et al. Marital conflict in older adults: endocrinological and immunological correlates. *Psychosom Med.* 1997;59(4):339-349.

24. Rohleder N, Schommer NC, Hellhammer DH, Engel R, Kirschbaum C. Sex differences in glucocorticoid sensitivity of proinflammatory cytokine production after psychosocial stress. *Psychosom Med.* 2001;63(6):966-972.

25. Kiecolt-Glaser JK, Malarkey WB, Chee M, et al. Negative behavior during marital conflict is associated with immunological downregulation. *Psychosom Med.* 1993;55(5):395-409.

26. Kiecolt-Glaser JK, Newton T, Cacioppo JT, MacCallum RC, Glaser R, Malarkey WB. Marital conflict and endocrine function: are men really more physiologically affected than women? *J Consult Clin Psychol.* 1996;64(2):324-332.

27. Burleson MH, Poehlmann KM, Hawkley LC, et al. Stress-related immune changes in middle-aged and older women: 1-year consistency of individual differences. *Health Psychol.* 2002;21(4):321-331.

28. Kiecolt-Glaser JK, Marucha PT, Malarkey WB, Mercado AM, Glaser R. Slowing of wound healing by psychological stress. *Lancet.* 1995;346(8984):1194-1196.

29. Malarkey WB, Kiecolt-Glaser JK, Pearl D, Glaser R. Hostile behavior during marital conflict alters pituitary and adrenal hormones. *Psychosom Med.* 1994;56(1):41-51.

30. Baum A, Cohen L, Hall M. Control and intrusive memories as possible determinants of chronic stress. *Psychosom Med.* 1993;55(3):274-286.

31. Elenkov IJ. Systemic stress-induced Th2 shift and its clinical implications. *Int Rev Neurobiol.* 2002;52:163-186.

32. Elenkov IJ, Webster EL, Torpy DJ, Chrousos GP. Stress, corticotropin-releasing hormone, glucocorticoids, and the immune/inflammatory response: acute and chronic effects. *Ann N Y Acad Sci.* 1999;876:1-11; discussion 11-3.

33. Elenkov IJ, Chrousos GP. Stress, cytokine patterns and susceptibility to disease. *Baillieres Best Pract Res Clin Endocrinol Metab.* 1999;13(4):583-595.

34. Ross M, Holmberg D. Recounting the past: gender differences in the recall of events in the history of a close relationship. In: Olson JM, Zanna MP, eds. *Self-Influence Processes.* Hillsdale, NJ: Lawrence Erlbaum Associates, Inc; 1990:135-152.

35. Collins BS, Hollander RB, Koffman DM, Reeve R, Seidler S. Women, work and health: issues and implications for worksite health promotion. *Women Health.* 1997;25(4):3-38.

36. Black PH, Garbutt LD. Stress, inflammation and cardiovascular disease. *J Psychosom Res.* 2002;52(1):1-23.

37. Lavoie KL, Miller SB, Conway M, Fleet RP. Anger, negative emotions, and cardiovascular reactivity during interpersonal conflict in women. *J Psychosom Res.* 2001;51(3):503-512.

38. Garfinkel M, Schumacher HR Jr. Yoga. *Rheum Dis Clin North Am.* 2000;26(1):125-132, x.

39. Cotter AC. Western movement therapies. *Phys Med Rehabil Clin N Am.* 1999;10(3):603-616, ix.

40. Devi NJ. *The Healing Path of Yoga: Time-Honored Wisdom and Scientifically Proven Methods That Alleviate Stress, Open Your Heart, and Enrich Your Life.* 1st ed. New York, NY: Three Rivers, Inc; 2000.

41. Raju PS, Prasad KV, Venkata RY, Murthy KJ, Reddy MV. Influence of intensive yoga training on physiological changes in 6 adult women: a case report. *J Altern Complement Med.* 1997;3(3):291-295.

42. Shannahoff-Khalsa DS, Beckett LR. Clinical case report: efficacy of yogic techniques in the treatment of obsessive compulsive disorders. *Int J Neurosci.* 1996;85(1-2):1-17.

43. Pandya DP, Vyas VH, Vyas SH. Mind-body therapy in the management and prevention of coronary disease. *Compr Ther.* 1999;25(5):283-293.

44. Malathi A, Damodaran A, Shah N, Patil N, Maratha S. Effect of yogic practices on subjective well being. *Indian J Physiol Pharmacol.* 2000;44(2):202-206.

45. Kamei T, Toriumi Y, Kimura H, Ohno S, Kumano H, Kimura K. Decrease in serum cortisol during yoga exercise is correlated with alpha wave activation. *Percept Mot Skills.* 2000;90(3 Pt 1):1027-1032.

46. Damodaran A, Malathi A, Patil N, Shah N, Suryavansihi, Marathe S. Therapeutic potential of yoga practices in modifying cardiovascular risk profile in middle aged men and women. *J Assoc Physicians India.* 2002;50(5):633-640.

47. Manocha R, Marks GB, Kenchington P, Peters D, Salome CM. Sahaja yoga in the management of moderate to severe asthma: a randomised controlled trial. *Thorax.* 2002;57(2):110-115.

48. Greendale GA, McDivit A, Carpenter A, Seeger L, Huang MH. Yoga for women with hyperkyphosis: results of a pilot study. *Am J Public Health.* 2002;92(10):1611-1614.

49. Weintraub A. The natural Prozac. *Yoga Journal.* 1999;November/December. Available at: www.yogajournal.com/health/133_12.cfm. Accessed May 7, 2004.

50. Telles S, Narendran S, Raghuraj P, Nagarathna R, Nagendra HR. Comparison of changes in autonomic and respiratory parametersof girls after yoga and games at a community home. *Percept Mot Skills.* 1997;84(1):251-257.

51. National Center for Complementary and Alternative Medicine. Yoga clinical trials. Available at: nccam.nih.gov/clinicaltrials/yoga.htm. Accessed May 18, 2004.

52. Stephenson K, Holiday D, Pinson B. Yoga for working women: results of a pilot study. *East Texas Medicine.* 2004;2(1):11-18.

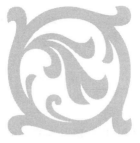

Chapter 4
Healing Images: Dreamwork, Cinematherapy, and Sandtray Therapy

Athena was the goddess of war and wisdom. This chapter is dedicated to women veterans, who in war and peace serve their country so valiantly, and to Terry Sparks, a chaplain and my former colleague at the veterans medical center in Amarillo, Texas. There are still women warriors; they fight battles every day. After leaving the military, many of these women feel forgotten and alone. They must face problems that many civilians could not imagine. Throughout her career as a military chaplain, Terry has provided guidance, solace, inspiration, and encouragement for the veterans who sought her help. She has awakened in those women other attributes of Athena to companion their valor and courage. She has helped them to heal, to face their fears, and to find a new purpose in civilian living.

I n ancient Greece, Athena was the primary symbol of feminine power in war and in peace. Images of the goddess, which abound even today, portray her strength, courage, and wisdom. Images and symbols remain as much a part of everyday life today as they were in ancient civilizations. They convey meaning without words and evoke recognition without language. For those reasons, they are tools useful in contemporary psychology and psychiatry. Symbols and images can reveal the source of conflict, fear, anger, and anxiety when words fail the patient.

Dreamwork, cinematherapy, and sandtray therapy are psychotherapeutic techniques that use images and symbols to enable insight and develop self-awareness. Those therapies help us to understand our role in conflict and to develop coping skills for resolving difficult situations. They enable the transformation that occurs when we awaken our innermost self and, in so doing, gain wisdom and inner strength.

Dreamwork

Dreams have a role in healing and nurturing the soul throughout life, and I have learned to appreciate the power of the messages they suggest. When I began my solo private practice in family medicine, I was well-prepared for most of the physical and mental illnesses that I treated but ill-prepared for the role of confidante. On several occasions, my patients revealed secrets to me that they felt could not be shared with another soul. Many of those confidences involved dreams that the patient thought too terrible, too strange, or too personal to discuss with a family member or friend. I found that hospitalized patients are particularly affected by troubling dreams and nightmares.

Because the number of my women patients who wanted to discuss their dreams increased, I decided to study dream therapy with a psychologist who was an expert in that field. I subsequently served as a staff physician at the local veterans administration hospital, where I became more active in assisting my patients with dreamwork.

Eventually, I helped to establish a dream therapy group for patients and employees at that facility.

The Hidden Messages in Dreams

Dreams are a symbolic language of images and archetypes that evoke an emotional response. They tend not to command specific action but rather to reveal questions and introduce possibilities. I encourage my patients to title their dreams and then to bring the dream imagery into their daily life as a sculpture or a drawing. If a patient has had a particularly inspiring, insightful, or confusing dream with a prominent image, I ask her to place an object representing that image on her bedside table, in her purse, or on her desk so that she can reconnect with the dream and reflect on its significance, its unique meaning, in her life.

Dreams often represent our gravest concerns and our greatest desires, as the following examples reveal.

The Floating Babies

One of my patients came to see me for her annual physical checkup. This patient had several health problems and needed to avoid future pregnancies. Because few contraceptive options were appropriate for her, she had decided that an intrauterine device (IUD) was the form of contraception that best met her personal and medical needs. At the time of her checkup, she had used an IUD for several years.

As I examined her, I noted that the IUD was in place and that it was causing no complications. After the examination, I explained my findings and asked whether she had any questions. She seemed unsettled and hesitant to talk. I waited. She then blurted out, "Can you take out my IUD today? It needs to come out!" Because she seemed distraught, I asked her if something had happened. She asked me if I understood how powerful dreams could be, and I nodded my head. At that point, she became tearful and stated that her dream — a recurrent nightmare — was too terrible to share. I assured her that I would not judge her because of its content, which she then related. In her vivid nightmare, hundreds of babies were floating in the sky. The patient was running on the ground as she tried to pull them down to earth and save them from decapitation by the sharp rotor blades of helicopters that were flying among them. Her rescue attempts were largely ineffective because there were so many helicopters and floating babies.

As we talked about the onset of those dreams and their details, she mentioned the comments of an acquaintance who had told her that IUDs were a form of abortion. He had called her a murderer for using that form of contraception. The patient and I then spent some time discussing her feelings and those comments, and I provided her with written medical evidence showing that an IUD does not cause any type of abortion. She was very relieved and departed reassured.

The Orphan Child
Another of my patients was strongly contemplating motherhood. She was a single, successful professional who felt a strong desire to have a child and was considering artificial insemination. Although she had almost completed the application process and had selected the donor profile, she remained ambivalent about the procedure. She had also considered adoption but wanted to avoid a long wait. As she struggled to make a choice, this patient had a vivid dream in which she approached a building that proved to be an orphanage. She knocked on the door and entered a room where a boy whom she had never met was sitting in a chair. He stretched out his arms to her and cried, "Mommy. *Mommy!*" At that moment, the

patient awakened, but the image of the boy in her dream remained very real. Later that week, a friend brought her information about an orphanage housing children in extreme need of adoption by a loving family. She decided to investigate. Several months later, she visited that orphanage and was introduced to a young boy who strongly resembled the child whom she had seen in her dream. She and this boy felt an instant affinity for each other; it was as if they had been reunited. She adopted him, which proved to be a joyful, life-changing experience for them both.

The Cheating Husband

One of my young married patients shared a troubling dream that recurred each week before her menstrual period. In the dream, she discovered signs that her husband was having an affair, and each dream involved his liaison with a different woman. In early dreams in the series, the signs of infidelity were subtle; her husband tried to hide his behavior. In later dreams, the "other woman" bragged openly about her relationship with the patient's husband, displayed gifts that he had given to her, and revealed intimate secrets that only the patient and her husband had shared.

After each such dream, this patient felt tremendous anger toward her husband, and her irritable mood persisted for several days. She had shared the content of one of the dreams with her husband, who had laughingly dismissed it as ridiculous. She told me that her marriage, while not troubled, was challenged by the usual worries and conflicts (finances, extended families, job stress, children) that young couples often experience. She valued her marriage and had no wish to end it. I then referred her to an excellent clinician for more in-depth counseling alone and with her husband. This patient eventually identified her deep-seated fear of intimacy, her lack of trust, and a fear of abandonment that was related to her own traumatic childhood. As a result of counseling that directed specific attention to nurturing the marriage and the patient's personal development, the dreams stopped.

The Physiology of Dreaming

Despite the scientific information that brain imaging and neurophysiologic assessment provide about sleep, expert opinion about dream activity differs. Dreams help us to access inner resources and resolve conflicts. When we dream, we make associations that are unlikely to occur when we are awake, and we explore problems too uncomfortable to confront in a conscious state.

Dreaming is associated with the rapid eye movement (REM) phase of sleep, and we usually dream more than 2 hours per night.[1,2] Patients who are repeatedly awakened during REM sleep or are sleep deprived experience fatigue; musculoskeletal pain; a decrease in infection-fighting substances in the bloodstream, which diminishes immune system function; an increased risk of obesity; greater numbers of the inflammatory markers that signal cardiovascular disease; and reduced performance on cognitive tasks.[3-6]

Newborns can sleep for as long as 18 consecutive hours, 12 of which are spent in REM sleep.[7] We must conclude that dreaming is essential to our health and well-being at any age.

Medications and Dreaming

Because some medicines affect dream content and the ability to dream, I always ask the patient about medication use before we begin dreamwork. Antidepressants, antipsychotics, analgesics (especially those that provide migraine relief), antianxiety medications, antiseizure medications, and various antihistamines can cause nightmares and alter REM sleep.[8] Some supplements, such as chromium, have been reported to affect dreaming.[9] Other drugs relieve sleep disturbances: Prazosin taken at bedtime has been helpful in reducing the incidence of nightmares and sleep disturbances in patients with posttraumatic stress disorder.[10]

Medical Conditions and Dreaming

Pregnant women often dream in alarming detail about topics related to labor, delivery, and the health of the baby; for example, having their "water" break in a grocery store, going into labor on an airplane, experiencing massive hemorrhaging, or having to undergo an emergency cesarean section. Some women dream that their baby has been born with a birth defect. Because dreams are symbolic, I reassure my patients that dreaming about such experiences does not mean that they will occur. Instead, troubling dreams can prepare the dreamer for the stress of pregnancy, labor, and delivery and even for the possibility that complications might occur.

In some of my premenopausal patients, a decrease in dreaming and less vivid dreams are caused by a hormone imbalance. The usual dreamlife of those patients is restored when their hormone levels return to a normal range. I have observed that terminally ill patients often dream more vividly in the weeks before their death. Dreams of travel (being in a train station or an airport, trying to purchase a ticket to go on a trip, traveling on a long journey by plane or car) often occur near the end of life.

Some dreams reveal health concerns. A case report from the Menninger Clinic described a patient who underwent mastectomy as treatment for breast cancer.[11] Three years later, she had a vivid dream in which a new cancer had developed. Her physician examined her and found cancer of the cervix. During the next 8 years, this woman experienced several dreams that accurately suggested the development of active disease, despite negative test results. This patient's case suggests that dreams can accurately signal an active disease process.

Results of a British study showed that patients with irritable bowel syndrome or inflammatory bowel disease dreamed significantly more often about events related to digestion than did those without such disorders.[12] Another study of patients with nocturnal migraine revealed that unpleasant dreams featuring misfortune or the expression of anger, apprehension, or aggression were associated with the onset of headache.[13]

Dreams and Gender

Research has revealed gender-related differences in the language that young adolescents use to describe their dreams. The most common nouns used by both genders in descriptions of dreams were "house" and "mother," and the most frequent verbs were "go" and "do."[14] The dream narratives of adolescent boys had a greater incidence of words such as "animal," "long," "enter," and "kill," and those of adolescent girls more often featured intransitive verbs and the words "teacher," "horse," and "put."

Another study revealed that adolescent girls 13 or 16 years of age experience more disturbing dreams than do adolescent boys of the same age.[15] The study also showed that the frequent occurrence of disturbing dreams is associated with anxiety in boys and girls as young as 13 years.[15]

In a Turkish study, nightmares were more prevalent in female college students than in male students, and the rate of traumatic childhood experiences was higher in nightmare sufferers.[16] Other research indicated that although sensory experiences in dreams are rare, women were more likely than men to recall the sensation of smell or taste in a dream.[17]

Dreams and Guidance

Some dreams reflect the dreamer's intuition, regardless of age. I have experienced the benefits of such a premonition in my own family, as the following example reveals:

The Knowing Child

One morning, my daughter, who was in kindergarten, seemed very out of sorts when I awakened her. She was agitated and distraught, which was very unusual. When I soothed her, she sobbed, "Please don't take me to school today. *Don't* take me to school today!"

Because she had not been exhibiting school-related anxiety and I was not aware of any change in that day's school routine, I thought that her fear might pass. I calmly asked her to get dressed while I prepared her favorite breakfast, which I hoped would cheer her up. When she came to the breakfast table, she had obediently dressed but was still pleading not to go to school. She sat at the table but did not eat a bite. At that point, I became concerned. I had planned to run errands with my toddler and then wait for my kindergartner for about an hour in a parking lot near the school. Because she was so upset, however, I felt that I should not take her to school, although I couldn't rationalize that decision and I did not want to change my plans.

I decided to call my husband to ask his advice. He spoke to my daughter, who kept repeating tearfully, "*Don't* take me to school today." He suggested that I allow her to stay home. When I told her of my decision, she immediately became calm, began playing, and then ate her breakfast. We spent a quiet, uneventful morning. My husband called to check on us midmorning, but nothing out of the ordinary had happened. That evening, we were shocked by the headlines in the local paper. That very day, an armed man had been wandering around the parking lot across from the school where I had planned to wait for my daughter. The police were alerted, and when they arrived at the scene, the man began firing at them. The police defended themselves and killed the shooter, whose death was ruled suicide by homicide after further investigation.

The Dolphin's Touch

Years ago, I had a profound dream of healing that was peppered with unusual and powerful images. In the dream, my husband and I were in the underground parking garage of a large building, possibly a hotel. A stranger approached us and shouted in Spanish for my help. I followed this person into a first-floor room with an Olympic-sized swimming pool in which no one was swimming. Three Hispanic women dressed in black were standing near the edge of the pool. They spoke to me heatedly in Spanish and gestured as they asked me to save someone who was drowning.

As I looked more closely, I saw a young girl about 12 years of age lying face up on the bottom of the pool. I jumped into the water and asked my husband to bring me a dolphin. I felt a strong sense of urgency and certainty about needing a dolphin to resuscitate the child. I waited in the water near her body for what seemed like a long time. As I waited, I felt compassion and sorrow, and I reassured the 3 women who stood crying near the edge of the pool.

My husband finally arrived with a dolphin, which he placed in the water near me. When I saw it, my heart fell; it was old and covered with scars. Its dorsal fin was torn and ragged. I doubted that it would be effective in resuscitating the girl. I pointed out its flaws to my husband and asked him to bring me a different one. He said that the old dolphin was all he could find and that I would have to use it.

Full of doubt and filled with desperation, I reached for the scarred dolphin and touched its body to the lifeless girl on the bottom of the pool. At the dolphin's touch, she opened her eyes, and I myself awakened. The dream was very real. Years later, it remains one of the most powerful experiences of my life. But my feeling when I awoke wasn't one of exhilaration and relief for having saved a child from dying. Instead, I felt frustrated and confused about the method that I had chosen to do so. Why, I asked myself, had I abandoned my medical training at such a critical time?

My instructor in dream therapy later helped me to interpret that dream at many levels. Like many of my physician colleagues, I had been taught that death is failure, that patients should never die on our watch, and that failed attempts at resuscitation are unacceptable. My teacher suggested, however, that I had realized that healing work and medical training are different types of interventions. I also knew, she said, that sometimes I needed to listen to the inner guidance that I possessed as a healer instead of simply carrying out technical protocols. I agree with her interpretation. Too often, we physicians forget that medicine is both an art and a science and that our professional heritage began not in the laboratory but at the bedside.

My teacher encouraged me to title my dream and then to bring its imagery into my daily life as a sculpture or a drawing of a dolphin. I did so, and that technique helped me to interpret the meaning of the dream in my personal and professional life. Now, if one of my patients has had a particularly inspiring, insightful, or confusing dream with a prominent image, I ask her to place an object representing that image on her bedside table, in her purse, or on her desk where she can touch and contemplate it.

Dreams and Healing
The Golden Handcuffs and Chronic Ovarian Cysts
One of my patients suffered from benign cysts on her right ovary. Ultrasonography showed that they were small and not worrisome medically, but they caused right-sided abdominal pain and discomfort during intercourse. I asked this patient to read the book *Women's Bodies, Women's Wisdom: Creating Physical and Emotional Health and Healing* (Northrup C. New York, NY: Bantam Books;1998), and to note the chapter on the "golden handcuffs syndrome," a mind-body connection in which women feel that they are locked into an unhealthful relationship or situation (especially those concerning finances) and that they have no way out. That syndrome is often noted in women who have ovarian cysts. My patient later said that the term "golden handcuffs" seemed especially applicable to her then because she was involved in several stressful situations that seemed beyond her control. Improved diet, medications, more exercise, and attempts at stress management did not alleviate her cyst-related pain, and surgical removal of the cysts seemed the only option for cure. At her next visit to my office, however, this patient was pain free. No medical or surgical intervention had been performed, but she described a dream that had immediately preceded her amazing recovery.

In the dream, she was lying on a comfortable bed. She felt very warm and secure, and she was peaceful and content. An angel surrounded by light and an array of muted colors then appeared, stood beside her, touched her abdomen and removed a ball-shaped crystal from her right side, comforted her, and disappeared. When the patient awoke, the pain in her right side was gone. It never recurred, nor did pain during intercourse.

The Child Who Died

I once provided medical care for a family that seemed to be perfect. I secretly hoped that my family and my own children would be as successful. The parents were both professionals. They were attentive to their needs as a couple and to the emotional, spiritual, and physical needs of their children (2 girls and a boy). They were intelligent, caring, and comfortable to be with. The children, who made good grades and were good athletes, were responsible, kind, and caring and had healthy peer relationships.

Eventually the girls left for college, and only the boy remained at home with the parents. One morning, the mother noticed that her son hadn't come downstairs for breakfast, so she called him. When he didn't answer, she went to his room and found him lying in bed. He was unresponsive, and she realized that he was dead. Autopsy revealed a minor congenital cardiac defect. He had died of sudden cardiac death, a condition in which the heart beats irregularly and then stops.

The mother became profoundly depressed. She lost more than 30 pounds and wore only dark colors. Pale and withdrawn, she became only the shell of the person she had been before her son's death. As her physician, I watched helplessly, knowing that I could not halt her emotional and physical decline. Each time I saw this patient, we would talk about her son's death, and she would repeatedly ask me whether she could have done anything to prevent it. What if she had checked on him during the night? What if he had had an asthma attack and wasn't able to call for help? What if he had died alone and in pain when she was in the house but not aware? She was filled with guilt, grief, and self-judgment. Her husband and daughters tried to assuage those feelings without success. One daughter eventually moved back home to provide additional support.

Three years after the boy's death, I was busy seeing patients when the receptionist told me that the mother was in my office and had asked to see me. I invited her to come in, and she entered the room smiling. Her eyes were bright; her skin, clear; and she seemed years younger. She was wearing a colorful summer sweater and a floral skirt. I was amazed and asked what had brought about this delightful change. She related the following dream, which she said had opened the path to healing.

In my dream, I was walking on a sidewalk in what seemed to be a small town in the mountains. I heard something, and when I looked up, I saw my son. He was driving a Jeep and stopped at the streetlight near where I was standing. He asked if I wanted a ride, and I jumped in. He looked very healthy and seemed peaceful and content. It was wonderful to sit next to him, to be so close to him. He asked how I was doing and told me that he was very happy. As we stopped at the final streetlight on the way out of town, he said that I would have to get out of the Jeep because he had to go on alone. I asked him where he was going, and he answered, "To *gan eden.*" He was very eager to get to his destination. I didn't want the stoplight to turn green, but it did, and I kissed him and got out of the Jeep. He continued on, and I stood on the sidewalk and watched the Jeep until I couldn't see it any longer.

When I awoke, I remembered the name of the place, *gan eden*, to which my son said he was traveling. It was a foreign name, and I asked my priest about its meaning. He said that it means "paradise" in Hebrew.

In my dream, the smell, feel, and nearness of my son was a healing balm for my heart, which had been aching so much to see him again. As I thought frequently about that dream, which was tremendously comforting, I was finally able to say good-bye and to find peace.

The powerful message in that dream freed my patient from her grief and enabled her to participate fully in life and to relate to others once again. That was a tremendous blessing for us all, because she is a highly gifted and very caring person.

Understanding Your Dreams
Perhaps this chapter has caused you to reflect on a vivid dream, a recurrent unpleasant dream, or a nightmare. The following suggestions about dream interpretation may be helpful:

• Write down your dream as soon as possible after you awaken. If you remember details of the dream during the day, add them to the description.

• Pay special attention to the images (male or female figures, numbers, symbols, animals) in the dream.

• Reflect on your attitude and associations with the dream content, and be especially aware of the text of recurrent dreams.

• Think of the dream as if it were a play or movie and not an actual occurrence.

- Learn about the common symbols evoked by the subconscious mind, which you can use to interpret your dream.

- Draw or paint the content of dream (this may be especially helpful for children).

- Join a dream group or work with a therapist who has expertise in dreamwork to gain additional insight about your dreams.

Cinematherapy

Several years ago, I began prescribing films as affordable, accessible, practical therapy to help patients better understand their intimate relationships, beliefs, and interactions with the outer world. I often suggest that a certain film be viewed by the patient alone or watched with a friend or family member.

Modern times call for modern solutions, and modern life pulls us in many directions. During a film, we can forgo the constant stimulation of pagers, cell phones, and e-mails for a 2-hour respite. Following the plot of a good movie requires us to focus on what is happening at that moment and prevents us from worrying about what we should be doing, didn't do, or don't want to do. Films transport us to a fantasy realm that provides brief relief from the overstimulation of a hectic lifestyle. A good selection of movies is readily available: Almost every town in America now has a video store. Public libraries often have a video section, and most of my patients can obtain their "movie prescription" at little or no cost.

Films are today's equivalents of fairy tales. They portray common archetypes (essential character types) that are present in each of us: the beautiful princess waiting to be rescued; the jealous and vengeful witch; the fire-breathing, destructive dragon; the courageous knight; the helpful, resourceful, or mischievous elves; the fairy godmother; and the evil queen. Sometimes we must awaken within ourselves a variety of archetypes to resolve a conflict or effect a change. When we watch a movie, we can explore the emotions of multiple characters from a distance while identifying the same feelings in ourselves.

Without confronting us, characters in a film teach positive and negative lessons by example. A film may serve as a catalyst for launching a dramatic change in behavior or lifestyle, or it might awaken new interests and provide fresh perspectives. Sometimes I recommend a film because I believe that the patient just needs to laugh. Themes such as romantic love, justice, transformation, hope, death, or the travails of a heroine's quest can awaken the Athena within a patient and liberate a passionate display of courage and strength. Our emotional and physical state and our life experiences also influence our response to what we see on screen.

> **Flicks in the Sticks**
>
> Flicks in the Sticks is a neighborhood outdoor movie club. Once each month, families meet for a potluck and a movie shown on a large screen designed and constructed by neighbors. This gathering of generations and friends offers time to rest, share, and reflect in the midst of the demands of modern living. The novelty of watching a movie under the night sky with neighbors is great fun; it's a reprise of the drive-in movie with the safety of home.

Responses to films are unique because each of us has a different level of emotional maturity, physical condition, and life experience. We all identify with movie archetypes, however, as the following examples demonstrate.

The Dominating Mother

One of my women patients suffered from migraines and bulimia. She confided in me during her office visits, and I suspected that her relationship with her mother contributed significantly to those disorders. This patient, a married woman in her 30s, had never become the adult child in her relationship with her mother. She was expected to be available at all times and was dominated by the overbearing demands and stern judgments of her mother, who constantly criticized my patient's choice of hairstyle, makeup, wardrobe, social activities, and friends, as well as her household proficiency.

After several visits to my office (including one in which her mother accompanied her), I asked this patient to watch the film *Like Water for Chocolate* with her husband. At her follow-up appointment, she confided that she had cried throughout the film as she began to realize how her own mother dominated and controlled her life. She also realized that most of her decisions were based on her mother's approval rather than on her own preferences or the needs of her family. My patient agreed to seek counseling, and over the next few months her migraines resolved and her bulimia improved. Although she found it very difficult initially to oppose her mother, she was eventually able to validate her own desires and tap into her strengths to gain emotional independence.

The Alcoholic Husband
Another of my female patients had multiple complaints (irritable bowel syndrome, migraines, fatigue, and a chronic stress-related skin condition). She was vague in her responses about her home life and marriage, and I didn't pressure her to reveal more than she was willing to share. During one appointment, she asked a few questions about the procedure of liver biopsy, which her husband was soon to undergo. When I inquired about those results at her next appointment, she said that the biopsy had revealed cirrhosis (a liver disease), and that her husband had been advised to stop drinking alcohol. I gently asked the patient about her husband's drinking. Her

answers strongly suggested that he was an alcoholic. She clearly wasn't ready to accept this possibility, so I asked her if she would be willing to see a few films by herself to explore the potential that her husband might have a drinking problem. She agreed to see the films *My Name Is Bill W* and *Under the Influence.*

During her return appointment, she stated that she had seen both films and had begun to suspect that her husband was indeed an alcoholic. I provided information about Al-Anon, an organization that offers counseling and support groups for family members of alcoholics. The patient attended her very first Al-Anon meeting that week. She eventually gained insight into her husband's alcoholism and associated emotional abuse. Over time, she developed greater inner strength and self-esteem, and her physical complaints gradually diminished.

Single-Mother Stress
One of my patients was a single mother who was completely focused on the physical and emotional needs of her chronically ill son. She was exhausted by everyday caretaking, frequent visits to physicians and emergency departments, and her child's hospitalizations, as well as the demands of a job that she didn't enjoy but that provided essential medical insurance. During her appointments, she appeared tired and worn-out. She was unable to talk about anything except her child. I tried to interest her in some concepts of self-care, but she resisted and said that she needed to use all available emotional and financial resources for her son and not for herself. I asked her to see the film *As Good As It Gets*, which portrays a single mother in a similar situation. During her next appointment, the patient stated that she had seen the film and had identified with the young mother. She realized that, like the featured character, she had no life apart from motherhood. She resolved to make some

changes and began to devote more time to self-care, which she so desperately needed.

My husband and I like to go to the movies. We have had a date night once a week for most of our marriage, and we usually see a film on that evening. Over the years, I have found cinematherapy to be as useful in my own life as it has been for my patients. I once served on location as the attending physician for Paramount Pictures when the movie *Leap of Faith* was being filmed. I hesitated before accepting that assignment because I was in my thirty-second week of pregnancy. I really didn't want 350 extra patients at that time, but my husband and I are great fans of Steve Martin, who starred in the film, and the opportunity to watch him in action was too good to miss. I provided medical care on the set, in trucks, and in the actors' trailers or apartments. Seeing the stars as patients with physical problems like those that afflict the rest of us deepened my appreciation of film making as a truly human art form.

I often suggest films from the following list as cinematherapy for my patients:

Girls and Adolescents
> *Whale Rider*
> *Ella Enchanted*
> *Legally Blonde*
> *Freaky Friday*
> *Drop Dead Fred*
> *Finding Nemo*
> *School of Rock*
> *Singin' in the Rain*
> *The Wizard of Oz*
> *October Sky*
> *Shrek* (2001 and 2004)
> *Footloose*

The Breakfast Club
Pretty in Pink
Mean Girls
The Kid

Young Adulthood

Shakespeare in Love
One Fine Day
The Preacher's Wife
Like Water for Chocolate
Erin Brockovich
As Good As It Gets
My Big Fat Greek Wedding
Broadcast News
Monsoon Wedding
Moulin Rouge
The Cider House Rules
Titanic (1997)
Good Will Hunting

Adulthood to Midlife

Lorenzo's Oil
Terms of Endearment
Steel Magnolias
The Joy Luck Club
It's a Wonderful Life
Unbreakable
The Horse Whisperer
Michael

Midlife and Beyond

Babette's Feast
Shakespeare in Love
Chocolat
Fried Green Tomatoes
Paradise Road (1997)
Cocoon

Something's Gotta Give
Gandhi
The Red Violin
Driving Miss Daisy
What Dreams May Come
Finding Forrester

Sandtray Therapy

Sandtray therapy is a psychotherapeutic technique based on the work of the Swiss psychologist and psychiatrist Carl Jung.[18] According to Jung, the subconscious mind secures the attention of the conscious mind by identifying certain objects as being very appealing or attractive, not because of their value or purpose but because they symbolize a unique and important issue. We are drawn to such objects, often without really knowing why. That principle is the basis of sandtray therapy: Examining our spontaneous choice of symbolic objects helps us connect with the issues they represent.

In sandtray work, the patient creates a "sandscape" by choosing miniature objects from a large selection offered by the therapist and arranging them in a small tray of pure, white sand. Water may also be offered for use in the sandscape. The patient guides the therapy session. He or she interprets the sandscape to the therapist, and in doing so often experiences intense feelings previously unidentified and unexpressed. When those emotions have been accessed and explored, healing can begin.

Patients with a chronic illness (headache, irritable bowel syndrome, recurring or unremitting pain), individuals at risk for or diagnosed as having a life-threatening illness, and people who are in transition or are contemplating a major life change benefit from sandtray therapy. It is also effective for those who have suffered severe emotional or physical trauma that is difficult to discuss. During an appointment, such a patient might present a long list of physical complaints such as headache, back pain, poor sleep, digestive problems, and a low energy level. When asked about issues such as relationships, self-esteem, workplace stress, or family dynamics, however, she might hesitate to respond or might reply "I don't know." or "I'm not sure." Sandtray therapy enables these patients to express aspects of profound trauma in a nonverbal way that involves no confrontation, as the following examples reveal.

Military Secrets
I once served as the medical director of women's health and employee health in the US Department of Veterans Affairs, where it was my honor to provide medical care for men and women veterans. Most of the female veterans after World War II had experienced physical or emotion trauma in the military in addition to domestic violence, divorce, substance abuse, and other psychosocial stresses. Many had difficulty expressing their deepest feelings about those events. After reading the book *Kitchen Table Wisdom: Stories That Heal* (Remen RN. New York, NY: Riverhead Books; 1997), I was inspired to offer sandtray therapy to those patients. Our director supported the idea, and our patients received it enthusiastically.

At the veterans healthcare facility, sandtray exercises were often conducted in private individual sessions by our pastoral counselor, who had been trained in that therapy. In those cases, I viewed each completed sandtray with the counselor and sometimes also with the patient. The sand-scape, like radiographs and laboratory test results, was a visible map of the patient's inner self that assisted me in making therapeutic choices as a physician.

At the start of each sandtray session, the patient and the counselor meditated together. The patient was then asked to select several objects, position them in the sandtray, and discuss the meaning of the objects and their arrangement. Some patients placed their objects in an exact pattern on the top of the sand; others partially buried them or scattered them randomly. At the conclusion of the session, each patient received a photograph of her sandtray and perhaps one of the objects to keep and reflect upon.

In one individual therapy session, a female veteran chose a tiny figure of a gorilla holding a globe on its shoulder. She later revealed that she suffered from chronic back pain and headaches and was highly stressed by caring for 2 family members, working full-time, and attending college classes. She felt that she had the weight of the world on her shoulders. After she had discussed her sandscape, she became more aware of the profoundly negative effect of stress in her life and began setting barriers and limits in response to demands on her time and energy.

Another patient chose a female figurine and partially buried it in the sand under an American flag. This veteran had experienced sexual trauma during military duty. During sandtray therapy, she was able to discuss that incident for the first time. The sexual assault had greatly affected her physical, mental, and spiritual health, and obtaining the additional information she provided was very valuable in her treatment.

Yet another patient arranged her items in a perfect diagonal, and each item that she selected (a rattle, a pacifier, a baby's shoe) was associated with an infant. This veteran suffered from chronic, severe migraines but had been unable to talk about the conflict that contributed to their onset. As she later revealed, she felt torn between the responsibilities of a very challenging career and the demands of new motherhood. Participating in the sandtray exercise helped clarify that association. She began exploring ways to create a flexible work schedule so that she could spend more time with her child.

At the veterans facility, we also used sandtray exercises as group therapy to build a sense of community and enable a deeper dialogue among individual patients. In those cases, the small tray was replaced by a child's plastic swimming pool filled with sand to accommodate all the objects selected during the session.

The dialogue that occurs during group sandtray exercises can also transform a workplace in which competition, backbiting, and emotional tension are the norm into a healthy, supportive environment. I once led a sandtray exercise for a group of women who worked together in a challenging environment. As one of the women selected her objects and placed them in the sandtray, she commented, "I don't know why I chose this clown; I hate clowns. When I was a girl at the circus, a clown scared me, and I haven't liked them since." Another woman in the group, a new employee, seemed affected by those words. After a few moments she leaned forward and said, "She chose this clown for me. I haven't been able to share this with you, but I am terribly upset about something at home, and the child who is causing the conflict collects clowns just like that figurine!" She then began to share the problem. The group supported her emotionally, and over the next few weeks they made a special effort to care for her. Like that new employee, far too many women remain silent about their problems instead of discussing them and asking for help.

Sandtray exercises were a very effective therapy at the veterans healthcare facility. In 1999, at the First Biennial International Conference on Spirituality, Health and

Healing, which was held at the University of Arizona in Tucson, Arizona, my staff and I presented our findings on that modality as an effective tool in the primary care of women veteran patients.[19]

Synchronicity

Some events are synchronous; their association is unexpected, although they have a shared theme. Synchronicity is often associated with sandtray exercises. Several years ago as I was leaving for a group sandtray session, my 5-year-old daughter thrust an object into my hand and said, "Here, Mommy; you will need this for the sandtray." I looked at the object — a black-and-silver plastic motorcycle — and questioned its relevance to the group of highly educated and sophisticated women who were participating in the exercise. Nevertheless, I placed it among the other miniatures. During the sandtray session, a middle-aged woman approached the display of objects and with some emotion reached for the motorcycle. As she placed it in the sandtray, she related a deeply personal experience to the group. She later thanked me for having offered that object and commented on how much relief seeing and touching it had brought her.

The techniques described in this chapter use symbols and images to unlock deeper issues that influence our ability to act, to progress, and to find peace. Sources for information about these valid therapies are listed below.

Suggested Reading

Hillman J. *The Dream and the Underworld.* New York, NY: Harper & Row, Publishers, Inc; 1979.

Rogers R, Michlin N, Bode CE. *Mother-Daughter Movies: 101 Films to See Together.* New York, NY: St. Martin's Press; 2004.

Kelsey MT. *Dreams: A Way to Listen to God.* New York, NY: Paulist Press; 1983.

Sandford JA. *Dreams: God's Forgotten Language.* New York, NY: HarperCollins Publishers; 1989.

Sandford JA. *Dreams and Healing: A Succinct and Lively Interpretation of Dreams.* New York, NY: Paulist Press; 1979.

Savary LM, Berne PH, Williams SK. *Dreams and Spiritual Growth: A Christian Approach to Dreamwork.* New York, NY: Paulist Press; 1984.

Riffel H. *Your Dreams: God's Neglected Gift.* Lincoln, Va: Chosen Books Publishing Company, Ltd; 1982.

Clift JD, Clift WB. *Symbols of Transformation in Dreams.* New York, NY: The Crossroad Publishing Company/Herder & Herder; 1986.

Taylor J. *Dream Work: Techniques for Discovering the Creative Power in Dreams.* New York, NY: Paulist Press; 1984

Steiner R. *The Work of the Angels in Man's Astral Body.* Herndon, Va: SteinerBooks Anthroposophic Press; 1988.

Jung CG. *Memories, Dreams, Reflections.* New York, NY: Vintage Books; 1989.

References

1. Stickgold R. Finding the stuff that dreams are made of. *ScientificWorldJournal.* 2001;1:211-212.

2. National Institute of Neurological Disorders and Stroke. Dreaming and REM sleep. Available at: www.ninds.nih.gov/health_and_medical/pubs/understanding_sleep_brain_basic_.htm. Accessed May 29, 2004.

3. Carskadon MA. Sleep deprivation: health consequences and societal impact. *Med Clin North Am.* 2004;88(3):767-776, x.

4. Kundermann B, Krieg JC, Schreiber W, Lautenbacher S. The effect of sleep deprivation on pain. *Pain Res Manag.* 2004;9(1):25-32.

5. Meier-Ewert HK, Ridker PM, Rifai N, et al. Effect of sleep loss on C-reactive protein, an inflammatory marker of cardiovascular risk. *J Am Coll Cardiol.* 2004;43(4):678-683.

6. Moline ML, Broch L, Zak R. Sleep in women across the life cycle from adulthood through menopause. *Med Clin North Am.* 2004;88(3):705-36, ix.

7. Staunton H. The function of dreaming. *Rev Neurosci.* 2001;12(4):365-371.

8. Pagel JF, Helfter P. Drug induced nightmares — an etiology based review. *Hum Psychopharmacol.* 2003;18(1):59-67.

9. McLeod MN, Golden RN. Chromium treatment of depression. *Int J Neuropsychopharmacol.* 2000;3(4):311-314.

10. Raskind MA, Peskind ER, Kanter ED, et al. Reduction of nightmares and other PTSD symptoms in combat veterans by prazosin: a placebo-controlled study. *Am J Psychiatry.* 2003;160(2):371-373.

11. Horton PC. Detecting cancer in dream content. *Bull Menninger Clin.* 1998;62(3):326-333.

12. Lal S, Whorwell PJ. What do patients with irritable bowel syndrome dream about? A comparison with inflammatory bowel disease. *Dig Liver Dis.* 2002;34(7):506-509.

13. Heather-Greener GQ, Comstock D, Joyce R. An investigation of the manifest dream content associated with migraine headaches: a study of the dreams that precede nocturnal migraines. *Psychother Psychosom.* 1996;65(4):216-221.

14. Azzone P, Freni S, Maggiolini A, Provantini K, Vigano D. How early adolescents describe their dreams: a quantitative analysis. *Adolescence.* 1998;33(129):229-244.

15. Nielsen TA, Laberge L, Paquet J, Tremblay RE, Vitaro F, Montplaisir J. Development of disturbing dreams during adolescence and their relation to anxiety symptoms. *Sleep.* 2000;23(6):727-736.

16. Agargun MY, Kara H, Ozer OA, Selvi Y, Kiran U, Kiran S. Nightmares and dissociative experiences: the key role of childhood traumatic events. *Psychiatry Clin Neurosci.* 2003;57(2):139-145.

17. Zadra AL, Nielsen TA, Donderi DC. Prevalence of auditory, olfactory, and gustatory experiences in home dreams. *Percept Mot Skills.* 1998;87(3 Pt 1):819-826.

18. Bradway K. *Sandplay Bridges and Transcendent Function.* San Francisco, Calif: CG Jung Institute of San Francisco; 1986.

19. Stephenson K, Sparks T. Sand Tray Work in Patient Evaluation in a Primary Care Environment. Paper presented at: First Biennial International Conference of Spirituality, Healing, and Health; April 10, 1999; Tucson, Ariz.

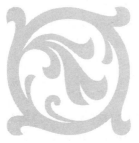

Chapter 5
The Value of Handwork

This chapter is dedicated to Sharon Wittenberg. Sharon is the proprietor of Purls, a comprehensive source of supplies for knitted projects, in Tucson, Arizona. Purls provides far more for its customers than beautiful yarns and excellent instruction in knitting. The store and its staff are dedicated to liberating creativity in women, building a sense of community, and reinforcing the great power of women working together. Through her guidance and inspiration, Sharon has taught many girls and women how to awaken the archetype of Athena, who is the goddess of handcrafts, and to find a center of inner stillness and peace in the midst of the turmoil of modern living.

A s our culture becomes increasingly automated and more technically driven, American women are literally losing touch. Store-bought toys and clothes are the standard, in contrast to the homemade items that were valued just a few generations ago. Has this convenience come at a high price? Have we rejected tasks that are intellectually and emotionally worthy in our efforts to save time? Women must respond to materialism and commercialism by reevaluating the value of handwork, which has an important role in ensuring physical and emotional health. For those reasons, I prescribe handwork projects such as knitting, weaving, cooking, or embroidery as therapy for many of my patients.

Value Across Cultures, Across Time

Working with the hands connects the intellect, emotions, and body, and healing occurs. In ancient times, some types of handwork were essential for survival. Today, women in some cultures view weaving, braiding, knitting, cooking, and other handwork as both practical and artistic, but many modern American women do not often engage in those activities. Several years ago, I took a knitting project with me to occupy my time while I was traveling to a medical meeting. At one point, the taxi in which I was riding slowed in bumper-to-bumper traffic, so I pulled out my knitting bag and began to work. As I knitted, the taxi driver, who was from East Africa, turned around to look back at me and shouted excitedly, "Ma'am, what are you doing?" Before I could answer, he repeated, "Ma'am, *what* are you doing?" I smiled and replied that I was knitting a handbag for my daughter. He asked, "Why don't you buy her a bag at the mall? Do you not have money?" I told him that I could indeed afford to buy a handbag but preferred to make one. He was incredulous. He then began talking excitedly about the clothes and other items that his mother had made for him when he was a child. He told me that during his 4 years in America "...this is the first time I have seen an American woman making something with her own hands for her children. Americans always go to the mall for their children's things. Your knitting makes me think of my mother. We were very poor, but she always made things for me and my brothers and sisters. I wish I still had them. You are a good mother. You love your children."

The Neurologic and Cardiovascular Benefits of Handwork

The brain develops at an exponential rate during childhood, which is a critical time in self-development for the introduction of handwork. Creating a handcrafted item encourages artistic individuality and creativity, and instruction in handwork is required in some of the most progressive current educational programs for children. Beginning in first grade, knitting, crocheting, woodworking, and other creative skills are taught in the elementary curriculum of the Waldorf schools, which form the largest group of independent private schools worldwide. Founded in 1919 by the Austrian scholar and philosopher Rudolf Steiner, the Waldorf curriculum is focused on developing each child's imagination and creativity in addition to proficiency in academic subjects.

Research shows that deficits in motor coordination like that used in handcrafts may portend future problems for some children. In 1999, a Finnish study documented the association between poor performance in handcrafts and sports during elementary school and the later development of schizophrenia.[1] No association of academic performance with later schizophrenia was noted.

The benefits of handwork also apply to adults. Neurologic research confirms that activities requiring the mobility and dexterity of certain fine-motor muscles (especially those of the hands) stimulate cellular development in the adult human brain.[2] Knitting, for example, involves sequencing, counting stitches, analyzing color use and patterns, and moving a thread or yarn repeatedly and deftly between the fingers and hands. Those fine-motor activities require the communication of the right and left halves of the brain through the corpus callosum, a band of millions of nerve fibers that is larger in women (perhaps because of their multitasking orientation) than in men.[2]

In 1995, a French study demonstrated that people 65 years or older who participated regularly in activities such as traveling, performing odd jobs, knitting, or gardening had a lower risk of subsequent dementia.[3] Knitting and gardening require complex brain functions (the ability to innovate, initiate, and integrate complex activities to attain a goal), and performing cognitively demanding activities correlates with improved intellectual functioning in older adults.[4-7] Dr. David Snowdon's "nun study" revealed that American nuns who lived in the same region and community and continued a lifelong participation in demanding intellectual activities after the age of 20 years were less likely to experience age-related dementia.[8] In addition to potential neurologic benefits, handwork produces cardiovascular benefits. While they are knitting, sewing, or crocheting, many women experience a whole-body relaxation response that is reflected in a slower heartbeat and respiration rate.[9]

Television viewing, however, is a relatively passive activity that engages more automatic brain processes, requires less intellectual focus, and provides no neurologic or cardiovascular benefit.[10] The relationship between television viewing and obesity in children and adults is well-documented. In a recent 6-year study, the television viewing habits of 50,277 women who ranged in age from 30 to 55 years were correlated with the health of those same subjects at the study conclusion.[11] The results showed that each 2-hour-per-day increment in TV viewing was associated with a 23% increase in obesity and a 14% increase in the risk of diabetes. Each 2-hour-per-day increment in sitting at work was associated with a 5% increase in obesity and a 7% increase in diabetes. However, each hour per day of brisk walking was associated with a 24% reduction in obesity and a 34% reduction in diabetes. The incidence of obesity and diabetes was highest in women who watched more than 40 hours of TV per week and lowest in those who watched TV for fewer than 6 hours weekly. Even sewing was shown to be of greater cardiovascular benefit than was passively watching TV.

I provide some of my patients with a "media prescription": the number of leisure hours per week that can be spent online, watching TV, or video viewing without increasing the risk of adverse health effects.

The Psychologic Benefits of Handwork

Many of my patients have said that handwork provides relief from emotional stress during periods of extreme turmoil. One couple for whom I provided care were expecting their first child. Because of financial hardship, the mother had not sought prenatal care until late in her pregnancy. During her physical examination, several health-related concerns were identified. The results of ultrasonography and other tests showed that the fetus had a birth defect incompatible with life and would die within hours after birth.

Many families presented with such bad news react with a combination of blame, guilt, isolation, and discord, but this couple responded differently. Because they were carpenters, they decided to craft a coffin of the finest wood they could afford. They designed it with great care and worked diligently to complete it before the anticipated date of the baby's birth. During the mother's long labor, they comforted each other with great emotional support, affection, and compassion. They prayed together. Their baby was born and soon died. Despite their grief, they took some solace from placing his body in the coffin that they had so lovingly made.

Healing Grace from Timeless Art

Focused concentration and physical activity create inner stillness that furthers contemplation and reflection.

From that emotional center of gravity, insight develops. For some women, handwork is a catalyst for problem solving. It enables them to access their imagination and express their creativity. The self-esteem, joy, and satisfaction that follow the completion of a practical, beautiful handwork project nurture the spirit. Many patients who feel overwhelmed, highly stressed, distracted, detached, or unable to relax and enjoy the pleasurable aspects of life gain a sense of self-worth, accomplishment, and pleasure from handwork of various kinds. They learn to use the power of sewing, beading, knitting, or crocheting to help cope with tragedy, enable physical and spiritual healing, and comfort themselves in times of trouble. It is a pleasure to watch their creativity and confidence unfold as the clinic staff admire their crafts and sometimes place orders and commission projects.

The Power to Cope

One of my patients related this poignant story of coping with tragedy:

Soon after my husband and I married, I became pregnant at twenty years of age. I was twenty-one when my son was born. During labor and delivery, which were very difficult, I was very scared, and I felt that no one was communicating with me. I was eventually given a gas anesthetic, which subdued my emotions. I then overheard the physician talking to my husband and mother. He asked, "Has this ever happened in your family before?" I was terrified about what was wrong with my newborn son. My husband reassured me; he told me that although the baby had been born with his fingers fused together, the doctors could correct the problem. I did not want to see or hold my baby, but the nurse gave me no choice. She thrust him into my arms, and to my surprise I was immediately filled with a strong love for my child and a desire to nurture and protect him. At that moment, I felt that there was no force great enough to have taken him from my arms against my will.

My husband and I were soon told that our baby had spina bifida occulta and a rare syndrome called oculodentodigital dysplasia. During the days that followed, I sometimes felt that having a defective child was my punishment from God or that my son was being punished for some unknown reason. The doctors thought that he was severely mentally retarded and would die before he was one year old. After he celebrated his first birthday, they predicted that he would die before he was three, but again they were wrong. We were often advised to put him in an institution, but we resisted. We knew that he would have to undergo many surgical procedures to improve his quality of life, but we were ready to provide him with that care and with our support.

When I was a young girl, my great aunt taught me to knit, but I had abandoned that hobby. I began knitting again while I was waiting in the hospital during the first of the forty-nine surgeries my son underwent before he was six years old. I found that knitting was soothing, relaxing, and calming. It helped me to cope with the long hours during my son's surgeries and at his bedside, and it became a very important source of relief from anxiety and grief. Once, as we waited at the hospital during a procedure, our car was stolen from the parking lot. When my husband reported the bad news, my first response was, "My yarn was in the car!" I remember panicking because I wasn't sure how I would cope without being able to knit for our projected two-week hospital stay.

Knitting has helped me to cope with the challenges that have occurred so often in my life. During times of emotional grief and turmoil, it helped me to find an inner strength. It gave me confidence in my creativity and a sense of accomplishment, pride, and self-worth. Those feelings contrasted sharply with the struggle of caring for my son on a daily basis.

Another of my patients also rejected physicians' recommendations to institutionalize her child, whose birth-related injury caused severe cerebral palsy and profound mental retardation. This woman began to crochet soon after her daughter was born, and she continues to do so. Now she crochets primarily at night because she must frequently care for her daughter, who sleeps only a few hours at a time. This patient gives her projects as gifts, and I am fortunate to have received several of them. Each time I see her needlework, I admire her grace and her enduring motherly love, and I marvel at her skill. When I am impatient with my own daughters' independence or overactive expression of creativity, I remember the projects that this patient so lovingly and patiently completed. That careful work, a product of respite from demands and intrusions, reminds me of the challenges faced by another mother and daughter, and my impatience is tempered.

The Power to Heal
A woman in my practice who loved to knit was an avid fan of a popular singer and actor. When she became aware that one of his tours would include a city near her home, she decided to knit a beautiful afghan to present to him at the concert. She worked tirelessly on a full-sized deep-scarlet afghan, and her children and grand-

children admired her progress. She joyfully worked at this task each day, squeezing in time to accomplish small amounts of knitting between her 2 jobs, and she completed the afghan a few months before the concert. One evening in the interim, a friend shared information about the progressive illness of a woman whom my patient did not know. This woman's condition had continued to deteriorate even though she had been examined and treated by the best physicians in the city. The hope of her recovery was slim.

This woman had young children. Before her illness, she had been a physically strong, vibrant, and energetically involved wife and mother. She eventually became so weak that her family placed a bed or palette for her in each room of their large home so that she could participate in family activities instead of becoming isolated and confined to one bed. At that stage of her illness, treatment was ineffective.

As she heard the plight of this unfortunate woman whom she had never met, my patient suddenly felt a strong impulse to give her the scarlet afghan. She was overcome with the intensity of this feeling and took the afghan to work the very next day, where she instructed her friend to give it to the woman who was so ill. That intense feeling and the urgency to act so selflessly were relieved when my patient parted with the afghan.

Some time later, she received a card of thanks for the gift. The recipient commented on the beauty of the blanket and emphasized how surprised she had been to receive such a gift from a stranger. She described a warmth that seemed to radiate from the afghan as she carried it with her from room to room and lay beneath it. Shortly thereafter, this woman's physical condition began to improve unexpectedly, without changes in her treatment regimen or other medical intervention. She was soon stronger and could participate in more household activities. I believe that the warmth emanating from the afghan was a healing force that became a bond between the 2 women. It came first from the soul of the artist, my patient; then from the artist's hands that had so lovingly knitted the blanket; and finally from the work itself. Handmade items are imbued with the energy of the artist who makes them. Many cultural totems or religious items are associated with providing protection or ensuring the well-being of the individuals who possess them.

Other patients who have surprised me by their willingness to engage in handwork are women with a connective tissue disease such as rheumatoid arthritis, lupus, or polymyositis. Those patients have given me many exceptional handmade items over the years, and I remain amazed at the beauty of their projects, which were completed despite the artists' increasing disability. I asked one patient with rheumatoid arthritis how she managed to crochet in spite of her infirmity. She said that her will to complete her projects and the comforting repetition of crocheting freed her from focusing on her pain and disability.

The Power to Comfort

An artist called "The Bear Lady" provides an unusual ministry based on the power that special objects confer. She makes teddy bears from the clothes of deceased loved ones to comfort surviving family and friends. For more than 30 years, she has worked year-round to fulfill requests for her handmade bears, which are crafted from a favorite shirt, suit, or dress once worn by the deceased. That very personal fabric evokes an immediate and powerful memory that sustains and comforts those who are grieving. The Bear Lady often receives cards or letters describing the solace that holding such a unique remembrance provides.

Several of my female patients who have profoundly disabled children also enjoy handwork. I had thought that group of women to be the least likely to engage in an additional task because of their already heightened physical and emotional demands. When I asked them why handwork was important to them, most smiled and said that their crocheting, knitting, or cross-stitching kept them from "going crazy." I now believe that for those women, handwork was spiritual work. Perhaps they felt guilt for having brought an "imperfect" child into the world, and the task of bringing forth a new creation from a skein of yarn, some cloth, or thread healed the spiritual wounds of self-judgement. As they worked with their hands, they could undo their errors and redo their work with a sense of success that was absent from their daily activities as caregiver for a seriously disabled child. Praise for the beauty of their handwork was a much-needed source of validation and recognition.

With each new piece of handwork, the artist further develops the skill of imagining a finished piece of art before it is even begun. This ability to imagine the future while living in the present and remembering the lessons of the past is also a spiritually nurturing practice. It helps us to develop a "spiritual eye" with which we can more clearly see ourselves and others in a forgiving, compassionate, and understanding way.

Prescriptions for Inner Peace

Handwork As Therapy

Research confirms the benefits of art therapy for those who are bereaved, for emotionally or physically abused children, for women with eating disorders or other emotional problems, and for those suffering from postsurgical pain.[12-20] As a family physician, I expand the definition of art therapy to include any activity that is not part of the daily family routine or work plan and that involves the use of materials, creativity, and imagination.

I began prescribing handwork for many of my patients after observing the benefits that it confers. I believe that projects such as knitting, weaving, sewing, and woodworking provide time for self-reflection that diffuses anger and hostility. It is better to furiously hammer, saw, cut, tear, knit, or stitch than to slam a fist through a wall or strike a child. Sometimes the sound of a sewing machine or the whir of power tools replaces the hostile words we want to speak. Instead of saying something that we might later regret, we can weave anger, resent-

The Beauty of Beads

Beaded jewelry is one of the oldest recorded forms of artistic expression. By 4000 BC, beads and the materials used to make them (agate, carnelian, jasper) were often used in commerce.[1] Between 3000 and 4000 BC, personal adornment with jewelry, including beads, was an indication of social status.[1] Five hundred years later, bead-making was a long-established art. The tomb of Queen Pu-abi in Mesopotamia (now Iraq), in the ancient city of Ur, has yielded some of the most beautiful beads ever discovered.[1] Dating from 2500 BC, they were made with superb craftsmanship from lapus lazuli, carnelian, gold, silver, and agate.

The beadwork of contemporary artisans is unique and beautiful in its own right. A friend recently described how her interest in beading brought unexpected benefits:

Several months ago, I dropped a favorite beaded earring down the drain. It was made with crystal and Bali silver from India, and I knew that finding another pair would be impossible. As I looked at the remaining earring, it occurred to me that I might be able to make a replacement. I decided to take a class in beading, and after learning the basics, I successfully re-made the earring that I'd lost. I was able to replicate it for a fraction of the cost of the original, and I found that beading was fun! The more I got into it, the more I enjoyed it.

At first, I wanted to work with natural stones like turquoise and amethyst. Now I also work with many other substances, such as crystal glass, gold, or silver. I learned to crochet with light-gauge gold-colored, silver, or bronze wire, which is very relaxing, and to work with a cabochon, which is a polished stone or piece of glass that can be wrapped with silver or gold wire to create a pendant, ring, or bracelet.

ment, and the desire to attack into our handwork, pulling the yarn so tight that our fingers turn white. Unraveling a row of knitting or ripping out a seam is better than shouting harsh words that cut to the soul and cause deep, lasting wounds. Throwing oneself into a project that commands all our attention often makes it possible to control or resolve powerful surges of anger or desperation.

The release of stress hormones and substances such as epinephrine, which occurs when we are agitated or angry, lowers the level of infection-fighting immunoglobulin A and increases respiration, heart rate, and blood

---

Having the ability to create a design and see it materialize before my eyes is very satisfying. It is instant gratification. Putting beautifully colored beads together and turning them into lovely works of art is also tremendous fun! I began to check out local craft stores, and I found some lovely beads there and on the Internet. Soon I was making other things like necklaces and bracelets. I realized that I could create beautiful things myself, and I took great satisfaction in that. There's definitely a therapeutic value to using your hands creatively instead of just to accomplish tasks in an office setting.

When I began working with beads, I was coming out of a situation that was very difficult for my family. My husband was in politics. He was involved in a psychologically bruising situation that affected us both. I had spoken with a counselor who told me that women are like sponges; they absorb all the bad things around them. Although I was not in the spotlight, I absorbed all the negativism that a bad political situation can generate. But when I sat down and began to make something, it was magical. Creating something beautiful with my own hands brought me a deep sense of fulfillment. Many of the bruised feelings began to evaporate for the first time in two years. Beading became a rewarding pastime; it was very healing. My artwork showed that I could actually **do** something; that I could accomplish something, even when the world was down on me, telling me that I couldn't do anything. But I could make a lovely piece of jewelry that would make other people happy. Beading is a great pastime that helps to fill some empty hours. Otherwise, I'd be sitting around just watching television.

Reference: 1. Dubin LS. *The History of Beads: 30,000 BC to the Present.* New York, NY: Harry N. Abrams; 1995:11-12.

pressure.[21] The physical effects caused by negative emotions eventually compromise the function of the cardiovascular system[22] and the immune system. In contrast, the repetitive, focused action required by handwork induces a sense of calm that dissipates stress and counteracts its harmful effects.

Children intuitively realize the value of releasing conflict through physical activity. One of my younger daughters recently seemed upset when she came home from elementary school. When I gently questioned her, she stated that she "didn't want to talk about it." Shortly thereafter, she asked me for a bowl and a piece of scrap paper, and I sensed that she was still upset. While I prepared dinner, she sat at the kitchen table and slowly and deliberately tore the paper into tiny pieces until she had filled the bowl. She then took the bowl, dumped the paper pieces into the trash, and returned the bowl to me. At that point, I observed a shift in her mood, and she was her usual self. She never discussed what had upset her, but she had resolved the matter. Children are wise in their willingness to use their hands; they easily embrace the mind-body connection that adults often abandon.

Cooking As Therapy
Cooking can also be used to sublimate negative or destructive emotions in a positive way. Have you ever "boiled with anger" and watched a boiling pot, all the while projecting your fury into the rolling water? Peeling potatoes, kneading dough, and slicing vegetables soothe painful emotions. The tactile sensations from hot water, cold water, steam, soft cloth, and cool metal soothe our heart and intellect. Cooking commands our attention, forces us to focus on accomplishing a task that brings us benefit, and diverts our thoughts from anger, rage, or grief. Figuratively placing such an activity between ourselves and the person who is the object of our wrath cre-

ates a temporary barrier that absorbs our anger and destructive thoughts. It allows time to pass until we are ready to renew the conflict in a more emotionally mature manner.

The Benefits of Timeless Tasks

As I knit an afghan for a new baby, I say a prayer for the mother and child who will receive it. I craft thoughts of hope for their future into the design as I complete each row. My knitting teacher in Tucson, Arizona, shared the story of a woman who had come to her store to select yarn for baby blankets. This woman said that she had just left her doctor's office after being diagnosed with terminal inoperable cancer. Her hope was to make blankets for the grandchildren she would not live to see. She attentively selected the yarn and patterns and deliberately chose this final knitting project to fill her last months.

Special Cases: Survivors of Extreme Violence

It has been estimated that by 2010, 30% of US military recruits will be female.[23] Women who serve their country in active warfare suffer differently from their male counterparts. Their hardships also differ from those of most female civilians. Women in the military often have fewer financial and social support resources than do most civilian women, and they are more likely to experience physical and emotion trauma.[23] One study indicated that 77% of US female veterans reported a lifetime history of violent assault.[23]

Research indicates that as the number of women in the military has grown, so has the number of cases of posttraumatic stress disorder (PTSD) in female veterans treated at Veterans Administration healthcare facilities.[24] A recent study showed that in 1998, women accounted for 20% of all US military recruits, and 48% of those women reported having been violently assaulted while they were in the military.[24] In contrast, 9% to 13% of civilian women screened in community-based studies reported violent assault during a similar period of time.[24] The development of PTSD in women veterans is strongly associated with lifestyle factors such as substance abuse, smoking, and domestic violence. In addition, female veterans with PTSD have a greater incidence of somatic distress, depression, and eating or panic disorders.[24]

In my clinical work with women veterans, I have provided care for a significant number of patients who suffered combat-related physical and sexual trauma, as well as domestic violence after their return to civilian life. When I provided outpatient care at a veterans healthcare facility for women in various stages of healing, I often advised my patients to start a project involving some type of handwork. Some women chose to make potholders; others began painting, woodworking, cross-stitching, or sculpting. They would bring their projects to their clinic visits, and it was a privilege for me to see and admire their work. Some patients even gave me their crafts as gifts, and I treasure them greatly.

As I worked with these patients, I realized that handwork often provided a diversion from their physical complaints. In other cases, self-expression through art brought forth a transforming self-discovery. Many of these women were unable to articulate their deepest feelings, but their emotions poured out through their hands into an art form. I noticed that those who completed a project gained a sense of mastery and competence, even if they felt overwhelmed by other aspects of daily living.

I have also treated male war veterans who experienced similar healing benefits from handwork. One such patient collected rusty nails, which he cleaned and converted into pocket-sized crosses that he enjoyed giving to other patients and staff. Each completed project was a tangible reminder of his survival, progress, and artistic ability.

Engendering the Will to Live

Handwork sometimes becomes a passion that strengthens the will to live. One of my women patients baked specialty cakes as a hobby. She glowed and responded enthusiastically when we discussed her interest during our first physician-patient encounter. At that time, she was widowed and in her late 60s. She had several chronic illnesses but was living independently and was an active community volunteer. At our next appointment several months later, however, I barely recognized her. She arrived for her appointment in a wheelchair. She was pale, weak, and withdrawn. Her spirit seemed broken. Her daughter, who had accompanied her, provided an account of her mother's travails.

My patient had experienced a health crisis and had undergone major surgery, after which severe complications requiring more surgeries had developed. She was then unable to care for herself and had become clinically depressed. She did not utter a word as her daughter shared this history and I performed my assessment. After writing her prescriptions, I kneeled in front of her as she sat in her wheelchair so that we were at eye level. I stated my prediction that she would recover and bake a cake in her own kitchen by Christmas day, which was 6 months away. Her expression brightened briefly, but she gave no verbal response.

Over the next several months, this patient's medical condition became more complicated as other life-threatening medical conditions were identified and treated. During each of her visits to assess her progress, we talked about her baking a Christmas cake. As autumn ended, her emotional and physical condition gradually improved, and she was again able to bake with the skill that she enjoyed before her illness. Baking became an ever-greater source of accomplishment and an affirmation of her recovery, and her Christmas cake was ready in time for the holidays.

How to Begin

I tell my patients that lessons in handcrafts and the initial materials required are the only expenses because friends, relatives, and acquaintances will begin to share yarn, materials, patterns, and their expertise. It's best to begin with a small project; a practical item that can be used, displayed at home or work, or given as a gift. A limited time each day or each week should be devoted to the project, which should be portable for those of us who travel frequently.

If you are interested in knitting and are fortunate enough to live in Tucson, Arizona, I highly recommend instruction at Purls, where excellent teachers provide affordable knitting lessons in a supportive atmosphere. Quilting and craft circles or guilds, seniors centers, and often the neighbor down the street are sources of instruction in handwork. Sometimes, a handcrafts group is a safe place in which women who are experiencing emotional trauma can express their feelings and find support. Often, group dynamics provides a new perspective in the process of recovery from trauma or loss.

Starting a project is the most difficult part; when you have begun, it is often hard to stop. The calendar is a great source of suggestions for projects, and birthdays and holidays provide inspiration and motivation. Some days, we may feel so overburdened that it seems easier to "zone out" on the couch in front of the television than to devote time to handwork. At times like those, it is better to persevere with the project. That quiet time can help you end even the most challenging day with a sense of peace, order, and accomplishment.

Resources for Handwork Projects

Boerens P, Durbano L, Steadman S, Allen McKKL. *The Encyclopedia of Two-Hour Craft Projects.* New York, NY: Main Street; 2003.

[No authors listed] *Home Made Best Made: Hundreds of Ways to Make All Kinds of Useful Things.* Pleasantville, NY: The Reader's Digest Association, Inc; 2003.

Wyman M. *Effectiveness by Design Online Catalog.* — A source of great knitting patterns in words and classic symbols. The patterns seem complex but are simple to complete. Available at: members.aol.com/mwbydesign.

Jaffke F. *Making Soft Toys.* Berkeley, Calif: Celestial Arts; 1981.

Jaffke F. *Toymaking With Children.* Edinburgh, Scotland: Floris Books; 2003.
— These wonderful books for children and adults provide instructions for making many items for children who are hospitalized or otherwise at risk.

Falick M, Hartlove C. *Kids Knitting. Projects for Kids of All Ages.* Muskogee, Okla: Artisan; 2003 — Although written for children, this is an enjoyable and informative book for all beginning knitters.

The Kid's Workshop is a program offered nationwide by Home Depot. Children 12 years of age or younger join a parent or guardian (2 children per adult) on the first Saturday of each month to build and complete a project (a soapbox derby car, a bird house, a kaleidoscope, etc). There is no charge for the workshop, and all materials (including an apron for each child) are free. Contact a local Home Depot for more information about the Kid's Workshop.

Large J, Carey D. *Festivals, Family and Food.* Gloucestershire, United Kingdom: Hawthorne Press; 1996 — When I'm stressed, overwhelmed, and can't come up with ideas on my own, this book has never failed me.

Warm Up America! Foundation — A tax exempt charitable organization that assists in the creation of afghan blankets by volunteers and distributes the blankets to the needy and homeless. Information is available online at: www.warmupamerica.com/home.html.

Purls, 7862 North Oracle Road, Tucson, AZ 85704, telephone: 888-377-8757 — An excellent source of knitting instruction, quality knitting materials, and superior service to customers.

Churches, synagogues, temples, and mosques; senior citizen centers; and community centers may host handwork groups or craft circles.

For a small fee, local colleges often offer courses in handcrafts.

Quilts 4 Cancer:
Helping to Provide Comfort for Cancer Victims
Joe McCauley

A national charitable organization whose members make quilts they donate to help comfort cancer victims is based in a Pahrump [Nevada] home. Barb Johnston started the organization, called Quilts 4 Cancer, with her husband, Jim, three years ago, a year after they moved [to Pahrump] from New York state.

"I developed cancer at the same time my mother was dying of breast cancer," Barb says. "I had seen other quilts-for-charities organizations, and I just decided that I wanted to do one strictly for people with cancer."

All of the quilts that Barb and some 20 other women volunteers make they donate to cancer victims through hospitals, chemotherapy centers and hospices. Barb says that quilts are practical items, which help to comfort anyone, especially anyone who has cancer and who may be taking chemotherapy treatments.

"We call them 'comfort quilts,' " Barb says. "If you can think of yourself having severe flu, say you're going through chemotherapy, you're going to get severe flu-like symptoms every week for nine months while you're getting your chemo. Having a quilt to put around you, it just gives you a little bit of warmth and comfort."

"Once the IV for chemo starts, it's like ice water going through your veins," Barb says. "You're cold, even on a hot day. Chilled. It's like instant flu. So, having a quilt to put around you is almost like a grandmother's hug. There's just something about it. It's just not the same as a blanket."

Most of the quilts that Barb and the Quilts 4 Cancer volunteers make are 40-by-60 inches in size, mainly because that size will fit into most standard home washers and dryers. Pillows, too, can be quilted.

"The end result is that people are comforted by the quilts, it doesn't matter what the reason was for making them," Barb says. "There's such a sense of accomplishment when you get a quilt done .... You just know that someone felt better for getting it. If I wasn't quilting, I don't know what I'd be doing."

For more information about or to donate to Quilts 4 Cancer, contact Barb Johnston at 775-751-5356 or Victoria Brazzle at The Quilted Dragon, 775-751-9033.

From the December 2003 Ruralite Magazine; Valley Electric Association; Pahrump, Nevada, edition; pages 4-5. Reprinted with permission from the author and publisher.

Joe McCauley is a freelance writer/photographer and director of member services at Valley Electric Association in Pahrump, Nevada. He is also the author of Puck Dreams & Other Stories *(Bloomington, Ind: Authorhouse; 2003), a book about 16 people who pursued their dreams.*

References

1. Cannon M, Jones P, Huttunen MO, et al. School performance in Finnish children and later development of schizophrenia: a population-based longitudinal study. *Arch Gen Psychiatry.* 1999;56(5):457-463.

2. Carlson NR. *Physiology of Behavior.* 7th ed. Boston, Mass: Pearson Allyn & Bacon; 2000.

3. Fabrigoule C, Letenneur L, Dartigues JF, Zarrouk M, Commenges D, Barberger-Gateau P. Social and leisure activities and risk of dementia: a prospective longitudinal study. *J Am Geriatr Soc.* 1995;43(5):485-490.

4. Hultsch DF, Hammer M, Small BJ. Age differences in cognitive performance in later life: relationships to self-reported health and activity life style. *J Gerontol.* 1993;48(1):P1-11.

5. Arbuckle TY, Gold D, Andres D. Cognitive functioning of older people in relation to social and personality variables. *Psychol Aging.* 1986;1(1):55-62.

6. Schooler C. Cognitive effects of complex environments during the life span: a review and theory. In: Schooler C, Schaie KW, eds. *Cognitive Functioning and Social Structure Over the Life Course.* Norwood, NJ: Ablex Publishing Corporation; 1987:24-49.

7. Dartigues JF, Gagnon M, Barberger-Gateau P, et al. The Paquid epidemiological program on brain ageing. *Neuroepidemiology.* 1992;11(suppl 1):14-18.

8. Snowdon D. *Aging with Grace: What the Nun Study Teaches Us About Leading Longer, Healthier, and More Meaningful Lives.* New York, NY: Bantam Dell Books; 2002.

9. Benson H, Kotch JB, Crassweller KD. The relaxation response: a bridge between psychiatry and medicine. *Med Clin North Am.* 1977;61(4):929-938.

10. Schooler C, Mulatu MS. The reciprocal effects of leisure time activities and intellectual functioning in older people: a longitudinal analysis. *Psychol Aging.* 2001;16(3):466-482.

11. Hu FB, Li TY, Colditz GA, Willett WC, Manson JE. Television watching and other sedentary behaviors in relation to risk of obesity and type 2 diabetes mellitus in women. *JAMA.* 2003;289(14):1785-1791.

12. Sexton H, Fornes G, Kruger MB, Grendahl G, Kolset M. Handicraft or interactional groups: a comparative outcome study of neurotic inpatients. *Acta Psychiatr Scand.* 1990;82(5):339-343.

13. Ferszt GG, Heineman L, Ferszt EJ, Romano S. Transformation through grieving: art and the bereaved. *Holist Nurs Pract.* 1998;13(1):68-75.

14. Bentensky M. *Self-Discovery Through Self-Expression. Use of Art in Psychotherapy with Children and Adolescents.* Springfield, Ill: Charles C Thomas Publisher, Ltd; 1973.

15. Tibbets T, Stone B. Short-term art therapy with seriously emotionally disturbed adolescents. *Arts Psychother.* 1990;17:139-146.

16. Davis CB. The use of art therapy and group process with grieving children. *Issues Compr Pediatr Nurs.* 1989;12(4):269-280.

17. Jones JG. Art therapy with a community of survivors. *Art Therapy.* 1997;14:89-94.

18. Lubbers D. Treatment of women with eating disorders. In: Landgarten HB, Lubbers D, eds. *Adult Art Psychotherapy: Issues and Applications.* Philadelphia, Pa: Brunner/Routledge; 1991.

19. Schimmel BF, Kornreich TZ. The use of art and verbal process with recently widowed individuals. *Am J Art Ther.* 1993;31:91-97.

20. Perlstein S. Really caring: why a comprehensive healthcare system includes the arts. *High Performance.* 1996;19(4):23-27.

21. Rein G, Atkinson M, McCraty R. The physiological and psychological effects of compassion and anger. *J Adv Med.* 1995;8(2):87-105.

22. Lavoie KL, Miller SB, Conway M, Fleet RP. Anger, negative emotions, and cardiovascular reactivity during interpersonal conflict in women. *J Psychosom Res.* 2001;51(3):503-512.

23. Dobie DJ, Kivlahan DR, Maynard C, et al. Screening for post-traumatic stress disorder in female Veteran's Affairs patients: validation of the PTSD checklist. *Gen Hosp Psychiatry.* 2002;24(6):367-374.

24. Kubetin SK. PTSD Prevalence in some female veterans at 22%. *Family Practice News.* 2004;38(8):64-65.

Chapter 6
Creating Hormonal Balance

This chapter is dedicated to the memory of John R. Lee, MD, a pioneer and expert in the clinical use of bioidentical hormone replacement therapy (BHRT) for women. Dr. Lee was a graduate of Harvard University and the University of Minnesota Medical School. He practiced family medicine for 30 years in northern California. While maintaining a busy clinical practice and a demanding schedule of lectures and speaking engagements, he conducted a variety of ongoing research projects on the effects of hormone therapy. Dr. Lee was the author of many books and articles on the interrelationship of hormones and women's health. He was passionate, forthright, and dedicated to illuminating the truth about the safety and efficacy of bioidentical hormones. Dr. Lee died October 17, 2003, of a heart attack. His Athenian zeal for justice and truth will be long remembered by the many physicians and researchers who were inspired, educated, and motivated by his work.

The Function of Hormones
Hormones regulate the activity of cells and tissues in various organs of the body. The balance of endogenous hormones (those produced by the body) is essential to good

health and a feeling of well-being. In women, various sex steroid hormones (estrogen, progesterone, testosterone) and steroid hormones (cortisol, dehydroepiandrosterone [DHEA], and dehydroepiandrosterone sulfate [DHEAS]) exert powerful effects throughout life. Those hormones are listed with comment below. They often form the basis for a diagnostic hormone profile, which is explained later in this chapter. Imbalances in the levels of sex steroid hormones and steroid hormones can profoundly influence health and quality of life, but therapies that restore hormonal equilibrium are affordable and available.

Estrogen[1-4] is an essential hormone that is produced in women primarily by the ovaries and adrenal glands. It is also formed by conversion from a precursor (a substance from which another usually more potent form is produced) that is stored in fatty tissue. There are 3 clinically significant types of estrogen: estradiol (E_2), which is the most potent estrogen; estrone (E_1); and estriol (E_3). Estrone, which is derived from an estrogen precursor stored in body fat, is the most prevalent estrogen found in women after menopause. Estriol, the most active estrogen during pregnancy, is produced from both estradiol and estrone. Estrogen receptors, or binding sites, are found throughout the human body. By receiving estrogen and rendering it available for physiologic function, receptors enable hundreds of estrogen-dependent functions to occur.

Estrogen stimulates the development of the breasts and reproductive organs and ensures their function. In the brain, it boosts the synthesis and function of neurotransmitters that affect sleep, mood, memory, libido, and cognitive factors such as learning and attention span. Estrogen decreases the perception of pain, preserves bone mass, and increases the level of high-density lipoprotein (HDL), the good cholesterol. It also preserves the elasticity and moisture content of the skin, dilates the blood vessels, and prevents plaque formation in blood vessel walls.

Progesterone[1,3,5-8] is manufactured primarily by the ovaries. Lesser amounts are produced by the adrenal glands, peripheral nerves, and brain cells. Progesterone ensures the development and function of the breasts and female reproductive tract. In the brain, it binds to certain receptors to exert a calming, sedating effect. It improves sleep and protects against seizures. Progesterone is a diuretic. It enhances the sensitivity of the body to insulin and the function of thyroid hormones. It builds bone and benefits the cardiovascular system by blocking plaque formation in blood vessels and lowering the levels of triglycerides. Progesterone also increases libido and contributes to the efficient use of fat as a source of energy.

Testosterone,[1] which is manufactured in women by the ovaries and adrenal glands, enhances libido and sexual response. It strengthens ligaments, builds muscle and bone, assists brain function, and is associated with assertive behavior and a sense of well-being. Both stamina and restful sleep are influenced by the level of testosterone. It has a protective effect against cardiovascular disease in both men and women.[9-13]

DHEA[1] is the forerunner of androgen and estrogen in the sex hormone pathway in women. It is manufactured primarily by the ovaries and adrenal glands; lesser amounts are produced in the skin and brain. DHEA is the most abundant circulating hormone. It provides protection against the effects of physical stress and inflammation. DHEA increases libido and sexual arousal. It improves motivation, engenders a sense of well-being, decreases pain, and enhances immune system function. Individuals with a low DHEA level have an increased risk of certain cancers.[14-16] DHEA facilitates the rapid eye movement

(REM) phase of sleep, enhances memory, and assists in maintaining normal cholesterol levels.[17-19] When enzyme action in the body adds a sulfate molecule to DHEA, the hormone DHEAS (a weaker form of DHEA) is formed.[20]

Cortisol[21,22] is manufactured by the adrenal glands. It regulates the immune response, stimulates the production of glucose, aids short-term memory, and helps the body adapt to stress by increasing heart rate, respiration, and blood pressure. The level of cortisol increases early in the morning to prepare the body to meet the demands of the day. It gradually decreases throughout the day and reaches its lowest point in the evening (a pattern known as "circadian rhythm").[21-25]

Xenohormones

Xenohormones[26] are not produced by the human body. They are contained in various environmental pollutants and chemicals (pesticides, herbicides, industrial chemicals, plastics, the byproducts of fuel consumption) and in meat and dairy products derived from animals treated with medications or hormones. Xenohormones are introduced into the body by exposure to the contaminants mentioned above. They may block the actions of hormones made by the body or mimic the action of the body's hormones by binding to receptor sites and sending messages that alter cell activity, just as "real" hormones would do.[26]

Exposure to xenohormones is thought to contribute to the high rates of breast cancer in industrialized countries.[27] For that reason, I advise my patients to minimize their exposure — and that of their children — to those substances. I also suggest boosting immune system function by creating hormone balance; eating certain foods[28] such as citrus, broccoli, cabbage, tomatoes, peppers, cantaloupe, strawberries, and cauliflower, which are high in carotene and vitamin C; exercising appropriately; and drinking adequate amounts of water, all of which may offer protection against the effects of xenohormones.

Hormone Interactions

The interactions of sex steroid hormones with steroid hormones are also important in creating hormone balance. Those types of hormones respond not only to the environment and messages from other hormones in the brain but also to each other.

Estrogens and progesterone exert opposing effects on breast tissue and in the tissue lining of the uterus. A balance in the amount of estrogens and progesterone results in normal physiologic function and activity, but an imbalance can cause symptoms such as abnormal uterine bleeding and may increase the risk of certain diseases such as breast cancer.[29-35] Some sex steroid hormones may undergo conversion; for example, testosterone can be converted into estrogen, and estrogens and testosterone can be converted from DHEA. Other hormones promote or block such conversions.[36,37] Hormones can also interact at receptor sites different from their own; for example, cortisol may bind to progesterone receptors. A woman who is producing too much cortisol in response to stress may thus experience the symptoms of a low progesterone level.[7,38]

The Importance of Thyroid Hormones, Sex Steroid Hormones, and Steroid Hormones

Thyroxine (T_4) and triiodothyronine (T_3), which are hormones produced by the thyroid gland, are essential for normal metabolism, the growth and repair of cells, the efficient use of food for energy, and the normal functioning of the nervous system. Certain thyroid diseases such as hyperthyroidism (an overactive thyroid) or hypothyroidism (an underactive thyroid) are much more common in women than in men. Cortisol, DHEA, testosterone, estrogens, and progesterone affect thyroid hormone activity and function.[39-41] Levels of sex steroid hormones and cortisol that are too high or too low can also affect the action of thyroid hormones, and those interactions may be associated with the development of cancer and infertility.[42-44]

The Value of a Hormone Profile

A hormone profile is a collection of test results that reveal hormone levels. The physician who orders the profile chooses the hormones to be analyzed according to the patient's symptoms. By reviewing the profile, the physician can detect imbalances caused by too much or too little hormone. Effective treatment can then be designed to correct those imbalances. I have used hormone profiles to guide treatment for the symptoms of menopause, premenstrual syndrome, female sexual arousal disorder, and polycystic ovary syndrome. Hormone profiles are also useful in identifying imbalances that contribute to a host of health problems such as fatigue, fibromyalgia, anxiety, depression, metabolic syndrome, migraine, seizure disorders, obesity, connective tissue diseases, thyroid disorders, asthma, irritable bowel syndrome, chronic pain syndromes, and sleep disorders.

A hormone profile must be interpreted in the context of the patient's current health status, medication use, stress level, menstrual cycle, diet, and exercise level. Although correlating the information in the profile with those factors is only moderately time-consuming, physicians and their staff are sometimes reluctant to devote time to that task. That is unfortunate, because a hormone profile provides women with important data about their health and hormone status and, when used to plan a treatment regimen, saves cost and improves the outcome of therapy.

In women, a baseline profile of estrogen, progesterone, testosterone, cortisol, and DHEAS should be first obtained when a woman is in her early 20s and every year thereafter. Hormone levels should be evaluated in girls or women of any age if their symptoms suggest a hormone imbalance. The information from that assessment can influence the patient's choice of diet and lifestyle, as well as future decades of healthcare planning. Obtaining a hormone profile should be a healthcare priority for every woman.

Signs of Hormone Imbalance

The proper balance of hormone levels is essential for well-being. In women, the symptoms of hormone imbalance are most often associated with excess or insufficient levels of sex steroid hormones (estrogen, progesterone, testosterone) or steroid hormones (cortisol,DHEA). The most-often prescribed drugs in the United States in 2003 (the sales of which ranged from $2.4 billion to $6.8 billion) were Lipitor, Zocor, Prevacid, Procrit, Zyprexa, Epogen, Nexium, Zoloft, Celebrex, and Neurontin.[45] In my opinion, it is possible that the primary diagnosis for many women treated with these costly, potent medications may be hormone imbalance.

The more frequently observed symptoms of hormone imbalance in women are featured in the Table. However, I have also noted uncommon symptoms of hormone excess or insufficiency that are not listed there. I encourage any woman with unexplained symptoms not mentioned in this chapter to consult a physician and to obtain a hormone profile.

Table. Symptoms and Health Risks of Hormone Imbalance in Women

Insufficient Estrogen and/or Progesterone[2,3,5,6,46-50]	Excess Estrogen and Insufficient Progesterone (Estrogen Dominance)[5,6,29-34,51-55]	Excess Testosterone and/or DHEA [9,15,56,57]
Hot flashes	Increased risk of breast cancer	Acne
Headaches	Breast tenderness	Increased risk of bulimia and anorexia
Vaginal dryness	Fibrocystic breast disease	nervosa
Incontinence	Weight gain (hips, waist, and thighs)	Disturbed sleep
Tearfulness	Irregular menstrual cycles	Increased risk of breast cancer and
Depressed mood	Bloating	heart disease
Sleep disorders	Heavy menstrual periods	High levels of triglycerides
Heart palpitations	Increased risk of blood clots	Increase in facial and body hair
Osteopenia or osteoporosis	Ovarian cysts	Loss of scalp hair
Impairment of short-term memory	Food cravings (eg, for sugar)	Increased risk of metabolic syndrome
Decreased clarity of thinking	Increased levels of triglycerides	Irritable mood
Night sweats	Decreased libido	Increase in abdominal fat
Fatigue	Irritability	Depression
Aches and pains	Increased risk of uterine fibroid tumors	Ovarian cysts
Dry hair and skin	Hypersensitivity	Increased risk of polycystic ovary
	Increased risk of postpartum depression	syndrome
	Anxiety	
	Mood swings	
	Symptoms of premenstrual syndrome	
	Headaches	
	Increased risk of gallstones	

Determining Hormone Levels

Hormonal balance is essential to good health for women of all ages. Unfortunately, the accuracy of the tests used to determine hormone levels varies widely. The 2 most prevalent types of testing for hormone imbalance are saliva testing, in which a small sample of the patient's saliva is analyzed to determine the levels of specified hormones,

Insufficient Testosterone or DHEA [9,10,58-63]	Excess Cortisol [21-23, 60,64-69]	Insufficient Cortisol [21-23, 60,64-70]
Decreased libido, sexual receptivity, and sexual pleasure	Increased risk of breast cancer	Fatigue
Low energy and persistent, unexplained fatigue	Acne	Food cravings (eg, for sugar)
Blunted motivation	Decreased libido	Lowered body temperature
Diminished sense of psychologic well-being	Increased risk of heart disease	Irritability
Hot flashes	Food cravings (eg, for sugar)	Body aches and pains
Increased risk of heart disease	Lowered body temperature	Heart palpitations
Body aches and pains	Loss of scalp hair	Increase in allergic reactions and chemical sensitivities
Depressed mood	Elevated levels of triglycerides	
Increased risk of dementia	Irritability, depression, or anxiety	
Osteopenia or osteoporosis	Increased risk of dementia	
Incontinence	Decrease in muscle mass and stamina	
Increased risk of rheumatoid arthritis	Thinning of the skin	
Vaginal dryness	Midbody weight gain (waist)	
Impairment of short-term memory	Fatigue	
Disturbed sleep	Sleep disorders	
Decreased clarity of thought	Osteoporosis or osteopenia	
Decreased attention span	Short-term memory impairment	
Thinning of the skin	Headaches	
Decreased muscle mass and stamina	Heart palpitations	
Increased risk of fibromyalgia	Increased risk of immune system dysfunction	
Accelerated aging		

DHEA, Dehydroepiandrosterone.

and serum testing, which is based on the analysis of a blood sample from the patient.

Saliva Testing

Saliva testing has been used in clinical research, including studies conducted at the National Institutes of Health (NIH) for more than 30 years.[71] Saliva testing has been available to practicing physicians for over a decade, and

Medicare and many insurance companies provide reimbursement for its use.

Over years of clinical practice, I have found that saliva testing is the most accurate measurement of the body's availability of the steroid hormones cortisol and DHEA and the sex steroid hormones estrogen, progesterone, and testosterone. Saliva testing correctly identifies the level of hormone at the cellular level (ie, the biologically interactive form of the hormone), in contrast to a serum (blood) test, which measures the level of hormone circulating in the bloodstream.[1,71-96]

Serum Testing

Most serum tests define the normal range of hormones very broadly, which is a distinct disadvantage to their use. After the patient's blood has been drawn, a portion of the blood sample (the serum) is used to measure hormone levels. Most serum testing measures the level of "free" hormone (the hormone that can easily enter the cell), the level of "total" hormone (the hormone attached to substances that carry hormones in the bloodstream), or a calculated combination of both free and total levels of hormone. It is not an accurate reflection of the bioavailable hormone (the amount of hormone that is active in organs and tissues). In addition, the results of serum testing are often inconsistent, especially if the hormone value indicated is in the low-normal range.[85-89, 96,97]

Many women whose serum test results are normal cannot understand why they continue to experience the symptoms of hormone imbalance. Saliva testing, however, provides a more exact range of normal results. Saliva tests reflect the amounts of hormones that are active within cells, which most accurately identifies the levels of sex steroid hormones and steroid hormones that are produced by the body or are active in the body when a patient is receiving hormone therapy.[71,72,74,75,79,80,82,85,90,91,93] At present, however, the levels of thyroid hormones can be measured only by serum testing or blood spot testing (see www.salivatest.com/provider/Blood_Testing.pdf).

Follicle-stimulating hormone (FSH) testing, which is a type of serum test, is another frequently used hormone evaluation. FSH directs the maturation of ovarian follicles and the release of estrogen. It also prepares the uterus for the changes that occur during the first half of the menstrual cycle. The FSH test is frequently used to determine the hormonal status of premenopausal patients who may complain of hot flashes, mood changes, or other symptoms listed in the Table. Several of my patients had been told by a former physician that their symptoms were not hormone-related because the result of their FSH test was in the normal range.

The FSH test should not be used as an accurate measure of sex steroid hormone production or an indication of reproductive status for most women, because the level of FSH fluctuates widely during the decade preceding menopause.[1,98] A properly conducted FSH test requires that blood be drawn 3 times at 60-minute intervals beginning precisely at 8:00 AM.[99] The FSH reference ranges are based on the average of those 3 levels, but I have found that the test is often performed improperly. In many cases, only 1 blood sample is drawn for evaluation, usually during an appointment with the patient's physician at time other than 8:00 AM. The vital clinical decisions about a patient's hormonal status and subsequent treatment are usually based on the results of that single test. Many patients have told me that because their FSH level was in the normal range, their health concerns were dismissed by their former physician.

Saliva Testing Versus Serum Testing

In my early years of clinical practice, I was frequently frustrated with the inaccuracy of serum testing, the results of which often did not support my observations of patients. I changed my clinical approach, and at the time of this writing, I have ordered saliva tests instead of serum tests to measure hormone levels in thousands of patients. The accuracy of those results has greatly enhanced my diagnostic and therapeutic decision making. As an added benefit, a saliva test (ZRT Laboratory, Beaverton, Oregon) is much less expensive than a serum test, whether the evaluation of 1 or many hormones is required.

Saliva testing is easy to obtain and to perform. The patient can collect the sample at home or at work, thereby avoiding travel to a testing laboratory and the need for painful needlesticks. In addition, the stress induced by the venipuncture required to obtain blood for testing can significantly alter serum test results.[93] For that reason, a serum test may not accurately measure the patient's usual serum hormone level. Saliva testing, however, has not been shown to cause a stress response in patients.[93] Despite those advantages, saliva testing remains a greatly underutilized evaluation, and many women and their physicians are not yet familiar with its benefits.

When compared with serum testing, however, saliva testing does have some disadvantages. Proficiency standards mandated for serum testing by the Clinical Laboratory Improvement Act (CLIA), which ensures that testing procedures are performed according to professional standards and guidelines, have not been established for saliva testing. Laboratories that offer saliva tests may be certified by the CLIA, but that certification is based on the proficiency of the serum testing procedures also provided. In addition, performing saliva testing is technically demanding and challenging. As a result, the number of laboratories capable of offering that type of evaluation is limited.

Although some saliva test kits are advertised in women's magazines, I caution against their use. To ensure accurate results, the staff of a laboratory that performs saliva testing should include a certified medical director and a laboratory director. Proof of reliability and expertise in saliva testing should be provided, and knowledgeable medical and support staff should be available to consult with physicians and other women's health providers if necessary. The laboratory that I use for testing (ZRT Laboratory) provides hormone reference ranges for patients of all ages and for those treated with medications such as oral contraceptives or hormone replacement therapy (HRT), which could affect the test results. Fortunately, a multidisciplinary interest in women's health is increasing among healthcare providers, and some pharmacists and mental health providers are now including a hormone profile based on saliva testing as part of their routine care for women patients. For more information about saliva testing in your area, visit the following Web site: www.salivatest.com. ZRT Laboratory, which is listed in the resources section of this chapter, also offers blood-spot testing for the evaluation of thyroid hormone levels.

Many physicians who call me for information about saliva testing express uncertainty about using that method because "there is nothing about it in the textbooks." At their bidding and with an invitation from the senior editor of a highly distributed medical journal, I wrote a full-length manuscript titled "The salivary hormone profile in the clinical evaluation of the female patient." The manuscript was ultimately rejected by the senior reviewer of that journal, an "expert" obstetrician-gynecologist who read it before publication. He criticized the article as being of below-average relevance to primary care physicians, as including insufficient scientifically based information, and as being replete with unsupported statements of questionable accuracy. The junior reviewer, however, gave the content an exceptionally high rating and wrote, "This well-written manuscript provides very strong scientifically evidence-based information with relevant information that many practitioners are unlikely to be aware of in the context of the HRT scare. [It] presents the advances of measuring vs. guessing." The senior reviewer's status and negative pressure prevented the publication of that manuscript. I have submitted it to another journal so that this vital information can be disseminated to physicians who provide care for women.

The History of HRT

HRT has long been the standard treatment for managing the symptoms of menopause. In the United States, HRT research began in the 1920s. During that decade, investigators discovered that injecting spayed female mice with estrogens extracted from the ovaries of sows caused favorable changes in mouse vaginal tissue. The mice treated with estrogens also exhibited behavior characteristic of being in heat.[100,101] When commercial estrogen preparations became available in 1926, physicians began using those drugs to treat complaints related to menopause.[102]

In the late 1920s and 1930s in the United States, the symptoms of menopause were treated by twice-weekly intramuscular injections, administered in physicians' offices, of estrogens prepared from animal-ovary extracts.[100] The cost of twice-weekly injections of estrogens ($10,000 annually in current USD) was too expensive for most women, and the laborious process of extracting those hormones yielded only a small amount of estrogens.[100] In

1929, American researchers decided to pursue a more liquid source of estrogens that would facilitate hormone extraction. The urine of pregnant women was identified as an abundant source of those hormones. Clinical researchers sent their nurses to the homes of expectant mothers, who supplied gallon jugs filled with their urine for use as a source of HRT.[100] However, urine from pregnant mares was soon identified as a ready and endless source of estrogens; it was used to manufacture the drug Premarin (conjugated equine estrogens) for use as HRT. During the 1940s, treatment with Premarin was available and affordable for many women. Its use was limited to the treatment of menopausal symptoms.[4]

In the 1960s, the drug company Ayerst Laboratories launched a vigorous and highly successful campaign to market the long-term use of Premarin as a treatment to prevent the adverse effects of menopause, even in women with no menopausal symptoms.[4,101] That drug company supported Robert Wilson, MD, in his writing of *Feminine Forever*, a book in which the virtues of Premarin were extolled and menopause was described as "an estrogen-deficiency disease."[102]

Menopause is **not** an estrogen-deficiency disease. I have provided medical care for hundreds of postmenopausal women whose estrogen levels after menopause were in the normal range according to saliva testing, and more than half the postmenopausal women enrolled in my clinical research studies had a normal baseline level of estradiol. Using scare tactics or strategic marketing to bully or entice women into taking hormones is insensitive at the least and blatantly harmful at the most.

Feminine Forever sold more than 100,000 copies in 1966. Ayerst Laboratories then conducted selective research that demonstrated the benefits of treatment with

Premarin. The results of that research, which were published in respected medical journals and presented at medical conferences, influenced clinical and popular opinion for the next 40 years. Researchers and physicians who disagreed with those results were pressured to change their views.[101] Advertising techniques targeting physicians and women featured additional findings from selective research studies that further touted the benefits of Premarin. Women were told that its use as HRT delayed aging and prevented osteoporosis, Alzheimer's disease, and cardiovascular disease.[101] Although no rigorous research supported those claims, for almost 40 years US physicians encouraged women to take hormones like Premarin to ensure good health after menopause.

In the 1970s, a strong link between the prolonged use of HRT such as Premarin and the development of cancer of the uterus in postmenopausal women was identified.[103,104] In response to that research, the pharmaceutical industry developed the synthetic drug medroxyprogesterone acetate (MPA, Provera), which blocked the adverse effects of estrogen on the uterus. The approval of Provera (the "Pro" part of the drug Prempro [conjugated estrogens and medroxyprogesterone acetate]) by the US Food and Drug Administration (FDA) was based only on the activity of that drug in the uterus, and the promotion of HRT resumed. Research conducted in rhesus monkeys (the animal model of the menopausal human female) demonstrated that Provera adversely affected the coronary arteries, but little attention was given to those findings.[105,106]

In the 1980s and 1990s, the emphasis on using HRT to preserve femininity in postmenopausal women was replaced by the concept of HRT as prevention against a host of age-related disorders. Premarin and Prempro were presented in lay publications and in the medical literature as being protective against osteoporosis,

Alzheimer's disease, colon cancer, and cardiovascular disease in postmenopausal women. Both drugs were intensively marketed to physicians and female consumers. Pharmaceutical companies were successful in gaining endorsements from professional medical societies for the prophylactic use of Premarin and Prempro in postmenopausal women.[107] Prescription numbers for and sales of Provera and Prempro soared to their highest level in 2001.[108]

Advertising and HRT

As previously mentioned, advertising has played a key role in the clinical use of HRT in the United States. In the 1940s, menopause was equated with a disease state, and all menopausal women were defined as needing treatment to prevent the age-related effects of estrogen deficiency. Advertisements for HRT first appeared in medical journals at that time. The ads characterized menopausal women as witches or hags who, if treated with the appropriate HRT, were transformed into much younger-looking and substantially more attractive women.[109] That negative portrayal of postmenopausal women, which was supported by many in the medical community, led to an increased use of HRT in the United States.

In the 1960s, *Time* and *Newsweek* were among the magazines promoting HRT as a drug that helped menopausal women retain their youth.[110] American women were ready consumers for products that invigorated beauty, and gynecologists partnered with the publishers of women's magazines to promote HRT as a fountain of youth.[111] In contrast to the messages in those ad campaigns, research has revealed that in some cultures, women do not report experiencing menopausal symptoms, and no word for "menopause" exists in their language.[112] In various cultural groups in Thailand, India, Nigeria, and

Morocco, menopause is thought of as a transition that is anticipated positively.[112] As women are influenced by Western culture, however, menopausal symptoms are more likely to be reported.[112] According to one report, European physicians lamented that US women were much more likely to take HRT (and were more compliant when doing so) than were European women.[113] I believe that stereotyping by physicians and patients and gender-based marketing contribute to the high incidence of menopausal symptoms reported by US women and spur the subsequent disproportionate use of HRT. In the late 1990s, direct-to-consumer drug advertising contributed to the demand for treatment by featuring attractive female celebrities who extolled the benefits of HRT. In my opinion, the demand for HRT in the United States has been stimulated more by marketing, advertising, and sociopolitical forces than by scientific fact.

New Evidence About HRT: The Results of the Women's Health Initiative (WHI)

After the establishment of the Office of Women's Health at the National Institutes of Health (NIH) in 1992, women scientists, consumers, and other concerned healthcare professionals and lay groups demanded more rigorous study of the nationwide practice of prescribing HRT for postmenopausal women.[4] As a result, several well-designed studies of the long-term effects of HRT, including the Heart and Estrogen/progestin Replacement Study I (HERS I) and the Estrogen and Atherogenesis study, were launched. Neither of those studies showed that HRT was protective against cardiovascular disease.[114,115]

The Women's Health Initiative (WHI) trials, which are the largest randomized controlled trials in US history that have been devoted to the effects of HRT, were designed to assess the safety and efficacy of HRT in healthy post-menopausal women.[116] Study participants with a uterus received estrogen-plus-progestin (Prempro), and those without a uterus received estrogen alone (Premarin, which is derived from the urine of pregnant mares). Both trials were terminated early (the Prempro trial in 2002 and the Premarin trial in 2004) because the health risks of treatment outweighed the benefit of fewer osteoporosis-related bone fractures. The trials showed that in post-menopausal women with a uterus, treatment with estrogen-plus-progestin increased the risk for invasive breast cancer, coronary heart disease, stroke, and pulmonary embolism. In postmenopausal women without a uterus, treatment with estrogen alone had no effect on the risk for coronary heart disease but increased the risk for stroke and significantly increased the risk for blood clots.

It is worth noting that women with moderate-to-severe postmenopausal symptoms were excluded from participating in the WHI and that in none of the women studied were hormone levels monitored. It is possible that some of the subjects had normal estrogen levels at the start of the study, because their menopausal symptoms were mild when the study began. If that is the case, then treatment with Premarin or Prempro may have caused estrogen excess in those women and may have increased their incidence of adverse events such as blood clots, stroke, and breast cancer.

Despite the known risks of treating women with Premarin or Prempro, some US physicians have continued to prescribe those drugs for their patients. I have had physician after physician approach me after my lectures on prescribing bioidentical hormone replacement therapy (BHRT) to make statements such as "I'll keep prescribing Prempro. At least we have large clinical trials about it." Other physicians have said, "My wife has taken Premarin for years, and she hasn't had any problems, so I'll keep prescribing it for my patients." or "If I stop giving my patients Premarin, I'm afraid they'll get osteoporosis. We can take care of their breast cancer, but there isn't much we can do for osteoporosis." The attitudes of those physicians, who adhere to prescribing practices that are lucrative and comfortable for them, have contributed to the poor heath of countless of women patients. I hope that more clinicians will seek a science-based approach to prescribing HRT and that women will demand safe and effective treatment for the relief of their menopausal symptoms.

Actress and author Suzanne Somers provides an excellent example of that type of proactive health care. After her breast cancer was diagnosed, she refused treatment with tamoxifen against the advice of her physicians because she was concerned about the adverse effects from and health risks of that therapy. After researching various options, she chose to treat her menopausal symptoms with bioidentical hormone replacement therapy (BHRT), and she gives a full account of her decision to do so in her recently published book *The Sexy Years: Discover the Hormone Connection — The Secret to Fabulous Sex, Great Health, and Vitality, for Women and Men* (New York, NY: Crown Publishing Group; 2004).

One of my research patients, a postmenopausal woman in her 70s, recently said that she purchased copies of the book *What Your Doctor May Not Tell You About Breast Cancer. How Hormone Balance Can Help Save Your Life* (Lee JR, Zava D, Hopkins V. New York, NY: Warner Books; 2002) for her daughters and daughters-in-law. She said that she wanted them to have that vital information about hormones and to choose a path different from her own. She also purchased the book for her physician with the mandate that he should read it before her next appointment so that "he could more intelligently discuss hormone options." She stated that she had taken various hormones for 45 years because her doctor insisted that they were good for her health. She said, "I feel that I have been the victim of [his] unwillingness to think for himself instead of willfully following the direction of slick marketing by the drug companies."

Alternatives to HRT: Testing, Not Guessing

When hormone imbalance is detected early and steps are taken to correct it, progression to disease states may be prevented. To correct a hormone imbalance, I use the "test-and-treat approach," which involves assessing the patient's hormone levels and then providing individualized treatment such as customized dosages of bioidentical hormones, if needed, and lifestyle and nutrition recommendations designed specifically for that patient. The test-and-treat approach is far superior to the "guess-and-treat approach" that I was taught in medical school and residency and that is still used by many physicians. In the guess-and-treat approach, the patient reports her symptoms and the physician guesses which hormones might be out of balance before prescribing a standard dose of a hormone. If, at the follow-up visit, the patient's symptoms have not improved or her condition has worsened, her treatment is changed to another preselected dose of conventional hormone therapy. After several episodes of treatment with different hormones or changes in dosage, a patient who reports no improvement is often treated with a drug to relieve anxiety or depression. If that therapy fails, she is usually referred to a psychiatrist or is told that "Your problems are in your head." or "There is no treatment left to offer." and is dismissed.

Unfortunately, the guess-and-treat approach is still far too common in clinical practice. Most physicians would never prescribe drugs such as the blood thinner warfarin (Coumadin) or cholesterol-lowering medications without monitoring the patient appropriately. They are, however, very willing to prescribe highly potent hormones that can induce harm, but they do not believe that monitoring the effect of treatment is important.

The Health Benefits of Treating Hormone Imbalance

The precise diagnosis of hormone imbalance can motivate women to change their diet and lifestyle. Regular exercise, stress reduction, and good nutrition can favorably affect hormone production and metabolism. Having normal physiologic levels of certain hormones enables many people to feel well enough to adjust their diet and lifestyle. For example, women with a low progesterone level often crave sugar or are fatigued. Eating sugar-rich foods produces a fleeting feeling of energy but (coupled with a lack of exercise) causes weight gain over time. When I prescribe progesterone supplementation for such patients, they crave sugar less and have more energy. They are therefore more likely to exercise, make better food choices, and lose weight.

I provide each of my patients with a copy of her hormone profile. This snapshot of hormone status confirms that the patient's symptoms have a physiologic cause and can be used to educate spouses and children about the nutritional and lifestyle changes that will benefit the patient. One woman in my care stated that her hormone profile was the topic of conversation during dinner on the day of her follow-up appointment. When she showed her test results to her family, her son commented, "Gee, Mom, you're hormone-free, just like the chicken that you buy at the market." This patient's spouse and children had realized that her hormone levels, which were at rock bottom, contributed to her symptoms of extreme fatigue and decreased stamina. Their new understanding validated the patient's feelings and disproved the opinion that she "just wasn't trying hard enough."

BHRT

I prefer to prescribe bioidentical hormones, which are derived from plants, for my patients who need HRT. The safety of BHRT has been chronicled in many research studies.[117-124] In chemical structure and physiologic effect, bioidentical hormones are identical to those produced by human ovaries and adrenal glands. Because they fit into human hormone receptors more efficiently than do synthetic hormones, bioidentical hormones produce few adverse effects. BHRT offers a wide variety of therapeutic options and may be taken orally or sublingually, applied topically in creams or gels, or administered as vaginal suppositories (see the formulary at the conclusion of this chapter).

In summary, I have observed that treatment with BHRT produces greater benefit and fewer adverse effects than does treatment with synthetic hormone therapy.

How to Obtain BHRT

Bioidentical hormones must be prescribed by a physician and prepared by a compounding pharmacist in a dosage customized for each patient. For example, some patients may require progesterone and testosterone, but others may need a different combination of hormones. Each prescription is individualized according to the patient's unique medical needs. The FDA has mandated guidelines for the preparation of compounded drugs, and the BHRT that I prescribe for my patients is manufactured and compounded in compliance with those guidelines.

Hormones used in BHRT include:

Bi-estrogen (Bi-Est), a combination of estriol and estradiol. From 50% to 80% of Bi-Est is estriol, which has been shown to protect against breast cancer in animal studies.[125,126] Estriol causes little or no stimulation to the uterine lining[117,120] and is clinically effective for the treatment of symptoms caused by estrogen deficiency, such as vaginal dryness and atrophy, painful intercourse, and urinary tract disorders (incontinence, frequent urinary tract infections). Estradiol relieves symptoms such as vaginal thinning and dryness. It decreases hot flashes and night sweats; improves mood, energy level, sleep patterns, memory, and cognitive function; and reduces bone loss and the risk of developing type 2 diabetes.[121,122,127-129] It also helps to lower blood pressure.[130]

Tri-estrogen (Tri-Est), a combination of 80% estriol, 10% estradiol, and 10% estrone. I have found that only a few women need supplemental estrone, which is the primary estrogen produced after menopause. Estrone is produced from hormone precursors in peripheral fat tissue, so I typically reserve its use for underweight women or those of low-normal weight. The saliva test can be used to measure levels of estradiol, estrone, and estriol to evaluate the patient's response to BHRT and need for treatment revision.

Progesterone, a hormone commonly prescribed for women with too much estrogen relative to the level of progesterone produced by the body. Progesterone minimizes the stimulating effects of estrogen on the uterus.[131] It enhances the beneficial effects of estrogen on coronary arteries, and when given alone or combined with estrogen, it may improve bone mineral density.[119] Progesterone improves sleep, may increase libido, acts as a diuretic, lowers blood pressure, and improves the insulin-glucose balance to facilitate blood glucose control.[6,7,32,122,123,132-134]

DHEA, which is prescribed for women whose hormone profile as determined by saliva testing indicates a low level of DHEAS. DHEA enhances libido, helps to build bone mass, lowers the levels of cholesterol and triglycerides, improves the sense of well-being, and increases alertness.[16-19,118]

Testosterone, which is prescribed for women deficient in that hormone. It improves libido, helps to build bone mass, improves mood and the sense of well-being, increases muscle mass and strength, lowers the levels of cholesterol and triglycerides, normalizes blood glucose levels, and decreases body fat.[9,124,135]

The Effect of Bioidentical Progesterone Cream on Menopausal Symptoms

Because of my interest in BHRT, I conducted a study of the short-term effect of topical bioidentical progesterone cream on menopausal symptoms; on the levels of substances in the blood that promote blood clots, heart disease, and stroke; and on the level of cortisol (which is associated with an increased risk of cardiovascular disease and breast cancer). Thirty healthy postmenopausal women participated in the study, which was conducted at a university medical center. When my colleagues and I began recruiting and enrolling patients, we found a high level of interest among women in the community. Some of those women stated that their physician had warned them about the dangers of progesterone cream and had advised them to continue taking Premarin or Prempro instead of participating in the study. Others said that their doctor had told them that progesterone cream was not biologically active and that the research study was a waste of time.

Despite those objections, we had great success in quickly recruiting the study participants. The postmenopausal women, who ranged in age from 43 to 74 years (median age, 57 years), were assigned to one of two therapies: treatment with either topical progesterone cream in a dosage of 20 mg daily or a placebo cream, which contained no hormone. Neither the subjects nor the researchers knew which preparation was being used. At the end of 4 weeks of treatment, the study participants used no hormones for 2 weeks. They were then assigned to treatment with the opposite therapy for 4 weeks. At the end of the study, the subjects were evaluated according to a menopause symptom scale and the results of serum and saliva testing.

At the conclusion of the 12-week study, we found that treatment with topical bioidentical progesterone cream produced the following results:

• Relief of menopausal symptoms.

• A **decrease** in cortisol levels in women with abnormally high levels of that hormone. This is important because a high level of cortisol in women is associated with an increased risk of cardiovascular disease, dementia, infection, and cancer.[67,68]

• No increase in inflammatory factors or clotting factors, in contrast to the effects of Premarin and Prempro. Treatment with those drugs has been associated with an increased risk of cardiovascular disease, stroke, and cancer.[116]

• No treatment-related adverse effects.

We submitted the findings of our study to the American Heart Association for presentation at their 2004 national conference, but our research was rejected without explanation. I have observed that studies on using BHRT to improve the health of postmenopausal women are of low priority to many medical institutions that conduct clinical trials and to organizations that offer research forums. Our motivated research team has submitted our study for consideration by another national society because we strongly believe that physicians and women need to know this vital information. We shall not give up!

Hormonal balance, then, is essential to health and well-being. HRT has been shown to relieve the symptoms of menopause, which in the Western world is often viewed as a difficult phase of life. However, recent scientific evidence has demonstrated that the HRT long thought to be beneficial imposes serious health risks on those who opt to use it. Healthful alternatives, such as modifications in diet and lifestyle and treatment with BHRT, are affordable and accessible. In all cases of medical treatment, however, women must ensure that their health status is assessed accurately and that the options they choose are safe. Only then can the benefits of therapy outweigh the risks.

Acknowledgements

The author would like to acknowledge those involved in her research study titled "The effect of topical progesterone on thrombotic, antithrombotic, inflammatory factors, neuroactive hormones, and menopausal symptoms in postmenopausal women": Carol Price, MN, RN, who superbly coordinated the project; John Stephenson, RPh, who graciously compounded and provided the placebo and progesterone cream; and Pierre Neuenschwander, PhD, and Anna Kurdowska, PhD, whose assistance was invaluable. Others who contributed to the completion of this project were: Barbara Pinson, MD; Douglas Stephenson, DO; Danita Alfred, PhD, RN; Agnieszka Krupa, PhD; Debra Mahoney, PhD, C-FNP; David Zava, PhD; Mary Bevan, MBA; Susan Sparks-Bauer; Debbie Fielder; Rick Carter, PhD; James Stocks, MD; and Nancy Creech, MN.

Suggested Reading

Wilson J. *Adrenal Fatigue: The 21st Century Stress Syndrome.* Petaluma, Calif: Smart Publications; 2001 — This book is especially useful for patients with cortisol excess or deficiency. The Web site (www.adrenalfatigue.org) contains several self-administered tests and information on the treatment of this hormonal disorder in the United States.

Gillson G, Marsden T. *You've Hit Menopause, Now What? 3 Simple Steps to Restoring Hormone Balance.* Calgary, Alberta: Blitzprint, 2003.

Northrup C. *Women's Bodies, Women's Wisdom.* New York, NY: Bantam Books; 1994.

Northrup C. *The Wisdom of Menopause.* New York, NY: Bantam Books; 2001.

McEwen B. *The End of Stress As We Know It.* Washington DC: Joseph Henry Press; 2002.

Vliet EL. *Screaming To Be Heard: Hormonal Connections Women Suspect and Doctors Ignore.* New York, NY: M. Evans and Company, Inc; 1995.

Lee JR, Zava D, Hopkins V. *What Your Doctor May Not Tell You About Breast Cancer. How Hormone Balance Can Help Save Your Life.* New York, NY: Warner Books; 2002.

Lee JR, Hanley J, Hopkins V. *What Your Doctor May Not Tell You About Premenopause. Balance Your Hormones and Your Life from Thirty to Fifty.* New York, NY: Warner Books; 1999.

Lee JR, Hopkins V. *What Your Doctor May Not Tell You About Menopause. The Breakthrough Book on Natural Progesterone.* New York, NY: Warner Books; 1996.

[No author listed] *Changing Your Life Through Understanding Your Hormones. The Seventh Woman's Visual Information Series.* (video; Silver Spring, Md: The Seventh Woman, Inc; [No year listed]. Available at: www.theseventhwoman.com — A visual information series about BHRT.

Resources

Professional Compounding Centers of America (PCCA), 9901 South Wilcrest Drive, Houston, TX 77099. Toll-free phone number: 800-331-2498; Web site: www.pccarx.com — Contact PCCA to locate a compounding pharmacist or physician with expertise in BHRT in your area or to arrange for continuing medical education for your staff.

International Academy of Compounding Pharmacists (IACP), PO Box 1365, Sugar Land, TX 77487. Toll-free phone number: 800-927-4227; Web site: www.iacprx.org — Contact IACP to find a compounding pharmacist in your area.

Wiler Professional Compounding Centers of America in Canada, 744 3rd Street, London, ON N5V 5J2. Toll-free phone number: 1-800-668-9453 (24 hours); Web site: www.wilerpcca.com — Contact Wiler PCCA to find a compounding pharmacist in Canada.

Rocky Mountain Analytical, Unit A 253147, Bearspaw Road NW, Calgary, Alberta T3L 2P5 Phone number: 403-241-4513; Web site: www.rmalab.com — Contact Rocky Mountain Analytical to obtain saliva testing in Canada.

ZRT Laboratory, 1815 NW 169th Pl, Suite 505, Beaverton, OR 97006. Phone number: 503-466-2445; Web site: www.salivatest.com — Contact ZRT Laboratory to obtain saliva testing and blood spot testing in the United States.

References

1. Speroff L, Glass RH, Kase NG. *Clinical Gynecologic Endocrinology and Infertility.* Baltimore, Md: Williams & Wilkins; 1994.

2. Huber J. Effects of sex hormones on connective tissue. In: Berg G, Hammar M, eds. *The Modern Management of the Menopause: A Perspective for the 21st Century.* Pearl River, NY: The Parthenon Publishing Group; 1994:377-380.

3. Smith SS. Hormones, mood and neurobiology — a summary. In: Berg G, Hammar M, eds. *The Modern Management of the Menopause: A Perspective for the 21st Century.* Pearl River, NY: The Parthenon Publishing Group; 1994:279-284.

4. Barrett-Connor E. Hormones and the health of women: past, present, and future. Keynote address. *Menopause.* 2002;9(1):23-31.

5. Finn DA, Gee KW. The significance of steroid action at the GABA-A receptor complex. In: Berg G, Hammar M, eds. *The Modern Management of the Menopause: A Perspective for the 21st Century.* Pearl River, NY: The Parthenon Publishing Group; 1994:301-314.

6. Dalton K. *The Premenstrual Syndrome and Progesterone Therapy.* 2nd ed. London, England: William Heinemann Medical Books; 1984.

7. Mahesh VB, Brann DW, Hendry LB. Diverse modes of action of progesterone and its metabolites. *J Steroid Biochem Mol Biol.* 1996;56(1-6 Spec No):209-219.

8. Lee JR. *Natural Progesterone: The Multiple Roles of a Remarkable Hormone.* Sebastopela, Calif: BLL Publishing; 1993.

9. Rohr UD. The impact of testosterone imbalance on depression and women's health. *Maturitas.* 2002;41(suppl 1):S25-S46.

10. Moller J, Einfeldt H. *Testosterone Treatment of Cardiovascular Diseases: Principles and Clinical Experience.* Berlin, Germany; New York, NY: Springer-Verlag; 1984.

11. Rosano GM, Leonardo F, Pagnotta P, et al. Acute anti-ischemic effect of testosterone in men with coronary artery disease. *Circulation.* 1999;99(13):1666-1670. Erratum in: *Circulation.* 2000;101(5):584.

12. Webb CM, McNeill JG, Hayward CS, de Zeigler D, Collins P. Effects of testosterone on coronary vasomotor regulation in men with coronary heart disease. *Circulation.* 1999;100(16):1690-1696.

13. Worboys S, Kotsopoulos D, Teede H, McGrath B, Davis SR. Evidence that parenteral testosterone therapy may improve endothelium-dependent and -independent vasodilation in postmenopausal women already receiving estrogen. *J Clin Endocrinol Metab.* 2001;86(1):158-161.

14. Lissoni P, Rovelli F, Giani L, et al. Dehydroepiandrosterone sulfate (DHEAS) secretion in early and advanced solid neoplasms: selective deficiency in metastatic disease. *Int J Biol Markers.* 1998;13(3):154-157.

15. Zeleniuch-Jacquotte A, Bruning PF, Bonfrer JM, et al. Relation of serum levels of testosterone and dehydroepiandrosterone sulfate to risk of breast cancer in postmenopausal women. *Am J Epidemiol.* 1997;145(11):1030-1038.

16. Casson PR, Andersen RN, Herrod HG, et al. Oral dehydroepiandrosterone in physiologic doses modulates immune function in postmenopausal women. *Am J Obstet Gynecol.* 1993;169(6):1536-1539.

17. Morales AJ, Nolan JJ, Nelson JC, Yen SS. Effects of replacement dose of dehydroepiandrosterone in men and women of advancing age. *J Clin Endocrinol Metab.* 1994;78(6):1360-1367. Erratum in: *J Clin Endocrinol Metab.* 1995;80(9):2799.

18. Legrain S, Massien C, Lahlou N, et al. Dehydroepiandrosterone replacement administration: pharmacokinetic and pharmacodynamic studies in healthy elderly subjects. *Clin Endocrinol Metab.* 2000;85(9):3208-3217.

19. Labrie F, Diamond P, Cusan L, Gomez JL, Belanger A, Candas B. Effect of 12-month dehydroepiandrosterone replacement therapy on bone, vagina, and endometrium in postmenopausal women. *J Clin Endocrinol Metab.* 1997;82(10):3498-3505.

20. Burger HG, Dudley EC, Cui J, Dennerstein L, Hopper JL. A prospective longitudinal study of serum testosterone, dehydroepiandrosterone sulfate, and sex hormone-binding globulin levels through the menopause transition. *J Clin Endocrinol Metab.* 2000;85(8):2832-2838.

21. Kendall J, Loriaux DL. Disorders of the adrenal cortex. In: Stein J, ed. *Internal Medicine.* 4th ed. St. Louis, Mo: Mosby-Year Book, Inc; 1994:1350-1361.

22. Selye H. *The Stress of Life.* New York, NY: McGraw-Hill; 1976.

23. Elenkov IJ, Webster EL, Torpy DJ, Chrousos GP. Stress, corticotropin-releasing hormone, glucocorticoids, and the immune/inflammatory response: acute and chronic effects. *Ann N Y Acad Sci.* 1999;876:1-11; discussion 11-3.

---

24. Vedhara K, Hyde J, Gilchrist ID, Tytherleigh M, Plummer S. Acute stress, memory, attention and cortisol. *Psychoneuroendocrinology.* 2000;25(6):535-549.

25. Scott LV, Salahuddin F, Cooney J, Svec F, Dinan TG. Differences in adrenal steroid profile in chronic fatigue syndrome, in depression and in health. *J Affect Disord.* 1999;54(1-2):129-137.

26. Krimsky S. Hormonal Chaos: *The Scientific and Social Origins of the Environmental Endocrine Hypothesis.* Baltimore Md: Johns Hopkins University Press; 2000.

27. Davis DL, Bradlow HL, Wolff M, Woodruff T, Hoel DG, Anton-Culver H. Medical hypothesis: xenoestrogens as preventable causes of breast cancer. *Environ Health Perspect.* 1993;101(5):372-377.

28. Jellinck PH, Michnovicz JJ, Bradlow HL. Influence of indole-3-carbinol on the hepatic microsomal formation of catechol estrogens. *Steroids.* 1991;56(8):446-450.

29. Nelson HD, Humphrey LL, Nygren P, Teutsch SM, Allan JD. Postmenopausal hormone replacement therapy: scientific review. *JAMA.* 2002;288(7):872-881.

30. Huang Z, Willett WC, Colditz GA, et al. Waist circumference, waist:hip ratio, and risk of breast cancer in the Nurses' Health Study. *Am J Epidemiol.* 1999;150(12):1316-1324.

31. Formby B, Wiley TS. Progesterone inhibits growth and induces apoptosis in breast cancer cells: inverse effects on Bcl-2 and p53. *Ann Clin Lab Sci.* 1998;28(6):360-369.

32. Mohr PE, Wang DY, Gregory WM, Richards MA, Fentiman IS. Serum progesterone and prognosis in operable breast cancer. *Br J Cancer.* 1996;73(12):1552-1555.

33. Nagata C, Shimizu H, Takami R, Hayashi M, Takeda N, Yasuda K. Relations of insulin resistance and serum concentrations of estradiol and sex hormone-binding globulin to potential breast cancer risk factors. *Jpn J Cancer Res.* 2000;91(9):948-953.

34. Liehr JG, Ricci MJ, Jefcoate CR, Hannigan EV, Hokanson JA, Zhu BT. 4-Hydroxylation of estradiol by human uterine myometrium and myoma microsomes: implications for the mechanism of uterine tumorigenesis. *Proc Natl Acad Sci U S A.* 1995;92(20):9220-9224.

35. Foidart JM, Colin C, Denoo X, et al. Estradiol and progesterone regulate the proliferation of human breast epithelial cells. *Fertil Steril.* 1998;69(5):963-969.

36. Schmidt M, Renner C, Loffler G. Progesterone inhibits glucocorticoid-dependent aromatase induction in human adipose fibroblasts. *J Endocrinol.* 1998;158(3):401-407.

37. Maurer M, Trajanoski Z, Frey G, et al. Differential gene expression profile of glucocorticoids, testosterone, and dehydroepiandrosterone in human cells. *Horm Metab Res.* 2001;33(12):691-695.

38. Kowalski WB, Valle RF, Chatterton RT Jr. Response of the primate secretory endometrium to subchronic hypercortisolemia. *J Soc Gynecol Investig.* 1997;4(3):152-159.

39. Levey GS, Klein I. Disorders of the thyroid. In: Stein J, ed. *Internal Medicine.* 4th ed. St. Louis, Mo: Mosby-Year Book, Inc; 1994:1323-1350.

40. Arafah BM. Increased need for thyroxine in women with hypothyroidism during estrogen therapy. *N Engl J Med.* 2001;344(23):1743-1749.

41. Soest R, Muller-Lissner S. [Clinical manifestation of adrenal cortex insufficiency during thyroid hormone substitution]. *Dtsch Med Wochenschr.* 1996;121(13):406-408.

42. Shering SG, Zbar AP, Moriarty M, McDermott EW, O'Higgins NJ, Smyth PP. Thyroid disorders and breast cancer. *Eur J Cancer Prev.* 1996;5(6):504-506.

43. Datta M, Roy P, Banerjee J, Bhattacharya S. Thyroid hormone stimulates progesterone release from human luteal cells by generating a proteinaceous factor. *J Endocrinol.* 1998;158(3):319-325.

44. Bispink L, Brandle W, Lindner C, Bettendorf G. [Preclinical hypothyroidism and disorders of ovarian function]. *Geburtshilfe Frauenheilkd.* 1989;49(10):881-888.

45. [No authors listed] *Family Practice News.* 2004;34(9):1.

46. Unger J, Cady R, Rarmer-Cady K. Migraine headaches, part 3: hormonal factors. *The Female Patient.* 2003;28(5):31-34.

47. DeMasi MA. Hormonally associated migraine. *The Female Patient.* 2004;29(7):30-36.

48. Almeida OP. Sex playing with the mind. Effects of oestrogen and testosterone on mood and cognition. *Arq Neuropsiquiatr.* 1999;57(3A):701-706.

49. Fink G, Sumner BE, McQueen JK, Wilson H, Rosie R. Sex steroid control of mood, mental state and memory. *Clin Exp Pharmacol Physiol.* 1998;25(10):764-775.

50. Smith SS. Activating effects of estradiol on brain activity. In: Berg G, Hammar M, eds. *The Modern Management of the Menopause: A Perspective for the 21st Century.* Pearl River, NY: The Parthenon Publishing Group; 1994:257-268.

51. Harris B, Lovett L, Newcombe RG, Read GF, Walker R, Riad-Fahmy D. Maternity blues and major endocrine changes: Cardiff puerperal mood and hormone study II. *BMJ.* 1994;308(6934):949-953.

52. Rodriguez I, Kilborn MJ, Liu XK, Pezzullo JC, Woosley RL. Drug-induced QT prolongation in women during the menstrual cycle. *JAMA.* 2001;285(10):1322-1326.

53. Beynon HL, Garbett ND, Barnes PJ. Severe premenstrual exacerbations of asthma: effect of intramuscular progesterone. *Lancet.* 1988;2(8607):370-372.

54. Backstrom T. Epileptic seizures in women related to plasma estrogen and progesterone during the menstrual cycle. *Acta Neurol Scand.* 1976;54(4):321-347.

55. Herzog AG. Intermittent progesterone therapy and frequency of complex partial seizures in women with menstrual disorders. *Neurology.* 1986;36(12):1607-1610.

56. Weber B, Lewicka S, Deuschle M, Colla M, Heuser I. Testosterone, androstenedione and dihydrotestosterone concentrations are elevated in female patients with major depression. *Psychoneuroendocrinology.* 2000;25(8):765-771.

57. Sowers MF, Beebe JL, McConnell D, Randolph J, Jannausch M. Testosterone concentrations in women aged 25-50 years: associations with lifestyle, body composition, and ovarian status. *Am J Epidemiol.* 2001;153(3):256-264.

58. Bachmann G, Bancroft J, Braunstein G, et al. Female androgen insufficiency: the Princeton consensus statement on definition, classification, and assessment. *Fertil Steril.* 2002;77(4):660-665.

59. Notelovitz M. Hot flashes and androgens: a biological rationale for clinical practice. *Mayo Clin Proc.* 2004;79(4 suppl):S8-S13.

60. de Bruin VM, Vieira MC, Rocha MN, Viana GS. Cortisol and dehydroepiandrosterone sulfate plasma levels and their relationship to aging, cognitive function, and dementia. *Brain Cogn.* 2002;50(2):316-323.

61. Ehrenreich H, Halaris A, Ruether E, Hufner M, Funke M, Kunert HJ. Psychoendocrine sequelae of chronic testosterone deficiency. *J Psychiatr Res.* 1999;33(5):379-387.

62. Apperloo MJ, Van Der Stege JG, Hoek A, Weijmar Schultz WC. In the mood for sex: the value of androgens. *J Sex Marital Ther.* 2003;29(2):87-102; discussion 177-179.

63. Jensen MD. Androgen effect on body composition and fat metabolism. *Mayo Clin Proc.* 2000;75(suppl):S65-S68; discussion S68-S69.

64. Vgontzas AN, Zoumakis M, Bixler EO, et al. Impaired nighttime sleep in healthy old versus young adults is associated with elevated plasma interleukin-6 and cortisol levels: physiologic and therapeutic implications. *J Clin Endocrinol Metab.* 2003;88(5):2087-2095.

65. Turner-Cobb JM, Sephton SE, Koopman C, Blake-Mortimer J, Spiegel D. Social support and salivary cortisol in women with metastatic breast cancer. *Psychosom Med.* 2000;62(3):337-345.

66. Sephton SE, Sapolsky RM, Kraemer HC, Spiegel D. Diurnal cortisol rhythm as a predictor of breast cancer survival. *J Natl Cancer Inst.* 2000;92(12):994-1000.

67. Elenkov IJ. Systemic stress-induced Th2 shift and its clinical implications. *Int Rev Neurobiol.* 2002;52:163-186.

68. Elenkov IJ, Chrousos GP. Stress, cytokine patterns and susceptibility to disease. *Baillieres Best Pract Res Clin Endocrinol Metab.* 1999;13(4):583-595.

69. Black PH, Garbutt LD. Stress, inflammation and cardiovascular disease. *J Psychosom Res.* 2002;52(1):1-23.

70. Wilson JL. *Adrenal Fatigue: The 21st Century Stress Syndrome.* Petaluma, Calif: Smart Publications; 2001.

71. Riad-Fahmy D, Read GF, Walker RF Salivary steroid assays for assessing variation in endocrine activity. *J Steroid Biochem.* 198319(1A):265-272.

72. Read GF, Walker RF, Wilson DW, Griffiths K. Steroid analysis in saliva for the assessment of endocrine function. *Ann N Y Acad Sci.* 1990;595:260-274.

73. Finn MM, Gosling JP, Tallon DF, Baynes S, Meehan FP, Fottrell PF. The frequency of salivary progesterone sampling and the diagnosis of luteal phase insufficiency. *Gynecol Endocrinol.* 1992;6(2):127-134.

74. Lu Y, Bentley GR, Gann PH, Hodges KR, Chatterton RT. Salivary estradiol and progesterone levels in conception and nonconception cycles in women: evaluation of a new assay for salivary estradiol. *Fertil Steril.* 1999;71(5):863-868.

75. Lu YC, Chatterton RT Jr, Vogelsong KM, May LK. Direct radioimmunoassay of progesterone in saliva. *J Immunoassay.* 1997;18(2):149-163.

76. Sumiala S, Tuominen J, Huhtaniemi I, Maenpaa J. Salivary progesterone concentrations after tubal sterilization. *Obstet Gynecol.* 1996;88(5):792-796.

77. Campbell BC, Ellison PT. Menstrual variation in salivary testosterone among regularly cycling women. *Horm Res.* 1992;37(4-5):132-136.

78. Dabbs JM Jr. Salivary testosterone measurements: collecting, storing, and mailing saliva samples. *Physiol Behav.* 1991;49(4):815-817.

79. Dabbs JM Jr. Salivary testosterone measurements: reliability across hours, days, and weeks. *Physiol Behav.* 1990;48(1):83-86.

80. Dabbs JM Jr, Campbell BC, Gladue BA, et al. Reliability of salivary testosterone measurements: a multicenter evaluation. *Clin Chem.* 1995;41(11):1581-1584.

81. Petsos P, Ratcliffe WA, Heath DF, Anderson DC. Comparison of blood spot, salivary and serum progesterone assays in the normal menstrual cycle. *Clin Endocrinol (Oxf)*. 1986;24(1):31-38.

82. Lipson SF, Ellison PT. Development of protocols for the application of salivary steroid analyses to field conditions. *Am J Hum Biol*. 1989;1:249-255.

83. Faddy MJ, Gosden RG, Gougeon A, Richardson SJ, Nelson JF. Accelerated disappearance of ovarian follicles in mid-life: implications for forecasting menopause. *Hum Reprod*. 1992;7(10):1342-1346.

84. Metcalf MG, Livesey JH. Gonadotrophin excretion in fertile women: effect of age and the onset of the menopausal transition. *J Endocrinol*. 1985;105(3):357-362.

85. Koefoed P, Brahm J. The permeability of the human red cell membrane to steroid sex hormones. *Biochim Biophys Acta*. 1994;1195(1):55-62.

86. Hiramatsu R, Nisula BC. Uptake of erythrocyte-associated component of blood testosterone and corticosterone to rat brain. *J Steroid Biochem Mol Biol*. 1991;38(3):383-387.

87. Sannikka E, Terho P, Suominen J, Santti R. Testosterone concentrations in human seminal plasma and saliva and its correlation with non-protein-bound and total testosterone levels in serum. *Int J Androl*. 1983:319-330.

88. McCracken JA, Schramm W, Einer-Jensen N. The structure of steroids and their diffusion through blood vessel walls in a counter-current system. *Steroids*. 1984;43(3):293-303.

89. Krzymowski T, Kotwica J, Stefanczyk S, Debek J, Czarnocki J. Steroid transfer from the ovarian vein to the ovarian artery in the sow. *J Reprod Fertil*. 1982;65(2):451-456.

90. Vining RF, McGinley RA, Symons RG. Hormones in saliva: mode of entry and consequent implications for clinical interpretation. *Clin Chem*. 1983;29(10):1752-1756.

91. Lo MS, Ng ML, Azmy BS, Khalid BA. Clinical applications of salivary cortisol measurements. *Singapore Med J*. 1992;33(2):170-173.

92. Swinkels LM, Ross HA, Smals AG, Benraad TJ. Concentrations of total and free dehydroepiandrosterone in plasma and dehydroepiandrosterone in saliva of normal and hirsute women under basal conditions and during administration of dexamethasone/synthetic corticotropin. *Clin Chem*. 1990;36(12):2042-2046.

93. Vining RF, McGinley RA, Maksvytis JJ, Ho KY. Salivary cortisol: a better measure of adrenal cortical function than serum cortisol. *Ann Clin Biochem*. 1983;20 (Pt 6):329-335.

94. Devenuto F, Ligon DF, Friedrichsen DH, Wilson HL. Human erythrocyte membrane. Uptake of progesterone and chemical alterations. *Biochim Biophys Acta*. 1969;193(1):36-47.

95. Levine H, Watson N. Comparison of the pharmacokinetics of crinone 8% administered vaginally versus Prometrium administered orally in postmenopausal women(3). *Fertil Steril.* 2000;73(3):516-521.

96. Miles RA, Paulson RJ, Lobo RA, Press MF, Dahmoush L, Sauer MV. Pharmacokinetics and endometrial tissue levels of progesterone after administration by intramuscular and vaginal routes: a comparative study. *Fertil Steril.* 1994;62(3):485-490.

97. Rosner W. Measurement of androgens: methods and pitfalls [The Endocrine Society Continuing Medical Education Web site]. Available at: www.androgensinwomen.com/index.php3?l=abstract#rosner. Accessed August 26, 2004.

98. Burger HG. Reproductive hormone measurements during the menopausal transition. In: Berg G, Hammar M, eds. *The Modern Management of the Menopause: A Perspective for the 21st Century.* Pearl River, NY: The Parthenon Publishing Group; 1994:103-108.

99. Bakerman S. *Bakerman's ABC's of Interpretive Laboratory Data.* 4th ed. Scottsdale, Ariz: Interpretive Laboratory Data; 2002:251-252.

100. Rothman SM, Rothman DJ. *The Pursuit of Perfection: The Promise and Perils of Medical Enhancement.* New York, NY: Pantheon Books; 2003:34-37.

101. Dukes MN. The menopause and the pharmaceutical industry. *J Psychosom Obstet Gynaecol.* 1997;18(2):181-188.

102. van Keep PA. The history and rationale of hormone replacement therapy. *Maturitas.* 1990;12(3):163-170.

103. Ziel HK, Finkle WD. Increased risk of endometrial carcinoma among users of conjugated estrogens. *N Engl J Med.* 1975;293(23):1167-1170.

104. Smith DC, Prentice R, Thompson DJ, Herrmann WL. Association of exogenous estrogen and endometrial carcinoma. *N Engl J Med.* 1975;293(23):1164-1167.

105. Miyagawa K, Rosch J, Stanczyk F, Hermsmeyer K. Medroxyprogesterone interferes with ovarian steroid protection against coronary vasospasm. *Nat Med.* 1997;3(3):324-327.

106. Miyagawa K, Vidgoff J, Hermsmeyer K. Ca2+ release mechanism of primate drug-induced coronary vasospasm. *Am J Physiol.* 1997;272(6 Pt 2):H2645-H2654.

107. Rothman SM, Rothman DJ. *The Pursuit of Perfection: The Promise and Perils of Medical Enhancement.* New York, NY: Pantheon Books; 2003:91-98.

108. Hersh AL, Stefanick ML, Stafford RS. National use of postmenopausal hormone therapy: annual trends and response to recent evidence. *JAMA.* 2004;291(1):47-53.

109. Rothman SM, Rothman DJ. *The Pursuit of Perfection: The Promise and Perils of Medical Enhancement.* New York, NY: Pantheon Books; 2003:56-57.

110. Houck JA. "What do these women want?": Feminist responses to Feminine Forever, 1963-1980. *Bull Hist Med.* 2003;77(1):103-132.

111. Rothman SM, Rothman DJ. *The Pursuit of Perfection: The Promise and Perils of Medical Enhancement.* New York, NY: Pantheon Books; 2003:74.

112. Flint M. Menopause — the global aspect. In: Berg G, Hammar M, eds. *The Modern Management of the Menopause: A Perspective for the 21st Century.* Pearl River, NY: The Parthenon Publishing Group; 1994:17-23.

113. O'Leary Cobb J. Why women choose not to take hormone therapy. In: Berg G, Hammar M, eds. *The Modern Management of the Menopause: A Perspective for the 21st Century.* Pearl River, NY: The Parthenon Publishing Group; 1994:525-533.

114. Hulley S, Grady D, Bush T, et al. Randomized trial of estrogen plus progestin for secondary prevention of coronary heart disease in postmenopausal women. Heart and Estrogen/progestin Replacement Study (HERS) Research Group. *JAMA.* 1998;280(7):605-613.

115. Herrington DM, Reboussin DM, Brosnihan KB, et al. Effects of estrogen replacement on the progression of coronary-artery atherosclerosis. *N Engl J Med.* 2000;343(8):522-529.

116. [No authors listed] Findings from the WHI postmenopausal hormone therapy trials. [Women's Health Initiative Web site]. Available at: http://www.nhlbi.nih.gov/whi/. Accessed August 26, 2004.

117. Yang TS, Tsan SH, Chang SP, Ng HT. Efficacy and safety of estriol replacement therapy for climacteric women. *Zhonghua Yi Xue Za Zhi (Taipei).* 1995;55(5):386-391.

118. Yen SS, Morales AJ, Khorram O. Replacement of DHEA in aging men and women. Potential remedial effects. *Ann N Y Acad Sci.* 1995;774:128-142.

119. Rosano GM, Webb CM, Chierchia S, et al. Natural progesterone, but not medroxyprogesterone acetate, enhances the beneficial effect of estrogen on exercise-induced myocardial ischemia in postmenopausal women. *J Am Coll Cardiol.* 2000;36(7):2154-2159.

120. Head KA. Estriol: safety and efficacy. *Altern Med Rev.* 1998;3(2):101-113.

121. Itoi H, Minakami H, Iwasaki R, Sato I. Comparison of the long-term effects of oral estriol with the effects of conjugated estrogen on serum lipid profile in early menopausal women. *Maturitas.* 2000;36(3):217-222.

122. Hargrove JT, Maxson WS, Wentz AC, Burnett LS. Menopausal hormone replacement therapy with continuous daily oral micronized estradiol and progesterone. *Obstet Gynecol.* 1989;73(4):606-612.

123. Dennerstein L, Spencer-Gardner C, Gotts G, Brown JB, Smith MA, Burrows GD. Progesterone and the premenstrual syndrome: a double blind crossover trial. *Br Med J (Clin Res Ed).* 1985;290(6482):1617-1621.

124. Shifren JL, Braunstein GD, Simon JA, et al. Transdermal testosterone treatment in women with impaired sexual function after oophorectomy. *N Engl J Med.* 2000;343(10):682-688.

125. Lemon HM. Estriol prevention of mammary carcinoma induced by 7,12-dimethylbenzanthracene and procarbazine. *Cancer Res.* 197535(5):1341-1353.

126. Lemon HM, Kumar PF, Peterson C, Rodriguez-Sierra JF, Abbo KM. Inhibition of radiogenic mammary carcinoma in rats by estriol or tamoxifen. *Cancer.* 1989;63(9):1685-1692.

127. Koloszar S, Kovacs L. [Treatment of climacteric urogenital disorders with an estriol-containing ointment]. *Orv Hetil.* 1995;136(7):343-345.

128. Sonni R, Bondi G, Travaglini S. [Presenile and senile vulvovaginitis. Topical hormonal treatment with estriol]. *Minerva Ginecol.* 1991;43(4):177-179.

129. Giuliani A, Concin H, Wieser F, et al. [Hormone replacement therapy with a transdermal estradiol gel and oral micronized progesterone. Effect on menopausal symptoms and lipid metabolism]. *Wien Klin Wochenschr.* 2000;112(14):629-633.

130. Seely EW, Walsh BW, Gerhard MD, Williams GH. Estradiol with or without progesterone and ambulatory blood pressure in postmenopausal women. *Hypertension.* 1999;33(5):1190-1194.

131. Moyer DL, de Lignieres B, Driguez P, Pez JP. Prevention of endometrial hyperplasia by progesterone during long-term estradiol replacement: influence of bleeding pattern and secretory changes. *Fertil Steril.* 1993;59(5):992-997.

132. Rylance PB, Brincat M, Lafferty K, et al. Natural progesterone and antihypertensive action. *Br Med J (Clin Res Ed).* 1985;290(6461):13-14.

133. Lee JR, Zava D, Hopkins V. *What Your Doctor May Not Tell You About Breast Cancer. How Hormone Balance Can Help Save Your Life.* New York, NY: Warner Books; 2002.

134. Plu-Bureau G, Le MG, Thalabard JC, Sitruk-Ware R, Mauvais-Jarvis P. Percutaneous progesterone use and risk of breast cancer: results from a French cohort study of premenopausal women with benign breast disease. *Cancer Detect Prev.* 1999;23(4):290-296.

135. Sherwin BB, Gelfand MM, Brender W. Androgen enhances sexual motivation in females: a prospective, crossover study of sex steroid administration in the surgical menopause. *Psychosom Med.* 1985;47(4):339-351.

Formulary for Bioidentical Hormone Replacement Therapy

Note: This formulary is a guide for patients. Each woman has unique responses and needs that should be considered by her physician and compounding pharmacist in the development of an appropriate therapeutic regimen.

Hormone	Suggested Dosage		Dosing Route and Frequency
Bi-Est (80% Estriol, 20% estradiol, or may be adjusted)	Capsule in oil	1.25 mg, 2.5 mg, 3.75 mg, 5.0 mg 5.0 mg	PO daily
	*Tablet	1.25 mg; 2.5 mg; 3.75 mg, 5.0 mg	PO daily
	Cream	0.125 mg/mL; 0.25 mg/mL; 0.375 mg/mL, 0.5 mg/mL	1 mL to skin daily or bid
Tri-Est (80% Estriol, 10% estradiol, 10% estrone)	Capsule in oil	1.25 mg, 2.5 mg, 3.75 mg, 5.0 mg	PO daily
	*Tablet	1.25 mg, 2.5 mg, 3.75 mg, 5.0 mg	PO daily
	Cream	0.125 mg/mL, 0.25 mg/mL 0.375 mg/mL, 0.5 mg/mL	1 mL to skin daily or bid
Testosterone	Capsule in oil	2.0 mg, 3.0 mg, 4.0 mg, 5.0 mg	PO daily
	*Tablet	2.0 mg, 3.0 mg, 4.0 mg; 5.0 mg	PO daily
	Cream	0.2 mg/mL, 0.3 mg/mL, 0.4 mg/mL, 0.5 mg/mL	1 mL to skin daily
DHEA	Capsule in oil	5.0 mg, 10 mg, 15 mg, 20 mg, 25 mg, 30 mg	PO daily
	*Tablet	5.0 mg, 10 mg, 15 mg, 20 mg, 25 mg, 30 mg	PO daily
	Cream	0.5 mg/mL, 1.0 mg/mL, 2.5 mg/mL	1 mL to skin daily
Estriol Vaginal Supp	Supp	0.5 mg, 1.0 mg, 2.0 mg	Per vagina at bedtime for 2 - 3 days, then 2 - 3 times each week
Testosterone Vaginal Cream	Cream	1%, 2%	Apply to vulva and vagina 2 - 3 times each week-
Progesterone	*Tablet	100 mg, 200 mg, 300 mg, 400 mg	Cycling: 100 - 200 mg on days days 1 - 9, then bid - qid on days 10 to start of menstruation Noncycling: 200 - 400 mg daily - bid
	Capsule in oil	25 mg, 50 mg, 75 mg, 100 mg	PO daily
	Cream	10 mg/mL, 20 mg/mL, 30 mg/mL, 40 mg/mL, 50 mg/mL	1 mL to skin daily or bid
	Vaginal supp	25 mg, 50 mg, 100 mg, 200 mg, 400 mg	1 per vagina daily
Triiodothyronine	Capsule	7.5 mcg	daily - bid
		15 mcg	daily - bid
Sildenafil 2%	Cream	Pea-size amount applied to clitoris	30 min before sexual activity daily

Pearls

Note: *Tablets are compounded as troches that are to be swallowed. They are prepared in MBK (fatty acid) base, which is manufactured by the Professional Compounding Centers of America (PCCA) (Houston, Texas). The tablets may easily be halved or quartered by the patient to permit flexibility in dosing. Estrogens, testosterone, and DHEA can be combined in capsules, cream, or tablets for dosing convenience and cost benefit. Progesterone may be combined with other ingredients as well, but progesterone used to treat a woman who has menstrual cycles should be administered alone because of the difference in dosages required during the first and second half of the menstrual cycle.

The creams are compounded in Cosmetic HRT base (PCCA). The oil capsules contain an oil manufactured by PCCA. The sildenafil is compounded in Cosmetic HRT base (PCCA) that is usually flavored. The vaginal suppositories are prepared in MBK (fatty acid) base (PCCA).

Women in their 30s and 40s often need higher dosages of progesterone, especially for the treatment of mood and cognitive symptoms. Some patients respond well to a combination of oral and topical dosing.

PO, By mouth; bid, twice daily; DHEA, dehydroepiandrosterone; supp, suppository; qid, 4 times daily.

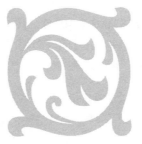

Chapter 7
The Power of Touch

The goddess Athena assisted the god Aesculapius in the healing arts, and the female archetype has been associated with nurturing and comforting those afflicted by illness, pain, or distress since antiquity. Florence Nightingale, who has long been honored for her contributions to contemporary health care, once stated that all women are nurses. I believe that the antidote for the ills of modern American life lies in the capable hands of women, whose dedication to family, friends, work, and society touches the lives of so many others.

This chapter is dedicated to the women who have devoted their life to medical missionary work and in so doing have touched the untouchable. Their dedication to healing, which requires great personal sacrifice, is an inspiration to all. My medical career has been guided and blessed by Sisters Helen Ann Collier, Barbara Ann Stowasser, Mary Schild, Eileen Mahoney, and Shawn Pickett, who have practiced their healing arts with Athenian courage throughout the world.

The Benefits of an Ancient Art

Touch has been considered a healing art since ancient times. The power of positive touch was deemed medical treatment in Ayurvedic texts and in the Ebers Papyrus, which is thought to have been written in Egypt around 1550 BC.[1,2] In ancient Greece, the touch of Aesculapius, the god of healing, was said to cure illness.[3] The laying on of hands is described in some Christian traditions as a method of healing the sick or conferring a blessing, and during the Middle Ages in Europe, the "king's touch" (the touch of a monarch) was sought as a cure for disease.[1]

Touch in the Animal Kingdom

Sentient living creatures respond to touch. According to some research, young animals that have been held, washed, cuddled, and physically nurtured experience better social and physiologic outcomes than do those deprived of such stimulation. Studies have demonstrated that the hormones oxytocin and prolactin, which affect behavior, and neuroactive substances such as dopamine, norepinephrine, substance P, and ß-endorphin, which are associated with relieving pain or physical distress, are released when rats, mice, and hamsters groom or touch each other.[4-11] The act of grooming has been shown to benefit the function of the immune and endocrine systems, to boost the physiologic response to inflammation, and to enable wound healing. Immune system dysfunction, hormone imbalances, behavior changes, and a diminished response to healing from wounding or trauma develop in rodents prevented from touching others and in those deprived of touch.[12-18] Research has shown that touch is also critical to the health of birds and dolphins.[19]

Saul M. Schanberg, MD, PhD, professor of pharmacology and cancer biology and professor of biological psychiatry at Duke University Medical Center in Durham, North Carolina, has devoted decades to research on the effects of touch.[20-22] Dr. Schanberg effectively demonstrated the association of touch with normal growth and development in animals. His landmark study showed that touch deprivation in mice pups caused a change in the expression (ie, the effect) of genes essential for survival. Despite access to adequate food, water, and housing, the pups separated from their mother 10 days after birth exhibited a dramatic deterioration of their physical state. Within 2 hours after maternal separation, a 40% decrease had occurred in the effect of various genes that direct growth and maturation. Other adverse events (for example, imbalances in the levels of hormones such as cortisol) also developed in those pups. The effect of reintroducing touch to the mice pups separated from their mother was then observed. A small paintbrush that had been dipped into water was used to stroke each tiny mouse. That tactile stimulation reversed the effects of maternal separation and reactivated the genes that determine growth and maturation.

Primatologist Jane Goodall, PhD, DBE, has demonstrated the importance of touch in higher primates.[23] In her work with the chimpanzees of Gombe Reserve in Tanzania, Dr. Goodall observed that grooming was an integral part of daily life and that even adult males sat together and groomed each other for several hours. When many of the chimpanzees were stricken with polio, one adult male that was paralyzed from the waist down dragged himself 60 yards to engage in a grooming session. If the chimpanzees wanted to be touched but were refused that interaction, they became agitated and expressed frustration.

Other research has confirmed the importance of touch in primate communities. In one study, macaques were isolated shortly after birth.[24] They received visual, auditory, and food stimuli but were deprived of tactile stimulation from other monkeys. As juveniles, they exhibited no intellectual deficits but demonstrated severe behavior problems such as social withdrawal, hyperaggression, and inappropriate sexual or parenting behavior. The length of isolation influenced the duration of troubled behavior: Macaques isolated for 3 months recovered from the deprivation, but those isolated for 12 months exhibited permanently inappropriate behavior.

Touch in the animal world, then, is not just about feeling good; it is essential to survival. Touching is a social activity that appeals to many animals, regardless of age or gender. Studies indicate that grooming occurs more frequently among animals in the wild than it does among those in captivity. It is an interaction that strengthens a vital social bond, and animals that do not form that bond are more likely to be caught by predators.[19]

The Power of Human Touch

All people, regardless of gender, age, culture, or heritage, benefit from positive tactile stimulation. Touch enables us to receive comfort and healing through the skin, which is the largest human organ. Our response to touch develops while we are in the womb. The moment we are born, we respond to tactile pleasure or pain and are primed to seek and receive physical contact.[25]

I have delivered many babies in my medical practice, and I have noticed that the first thing a newborn wants to do after exiting the womb is to touch. A tiny hand reaches out to grab something: the umbilical cord, my gown, my hand, or whatever can be reached in order to touch; to connect. This reflexive response to grasp is a sign of normal nervous system development, but I believe that it is also part of a newborn's innate willingness to bond and attach to a caregiver.

Touch has the same importance when we are dying. Although the sense of hearing, smell, or vision may diminish in the elderly or chronically ill, the sense of touch remains until the very end of life, except in people with certain rare diseases. I have never cared for a dying patient who did not want to touch another person or be held by someone during the final moments of life. There is a powerful connection between the emotions that sustain us and positive touch, which is essential to our well-being. For that reason, I prescribe touch therapy for many of my patients.

Cultural Differences in Touching

Evidence indicates that Americans have fewer positive touch interactions than do individuals in many other cultures. According to one study, adolescents were observed at McDonald's restaurants in Paris and Miami to determine their frequency of touching and aggression during peer interactions.[26] The American adolescents spent more time self-touching and were more verbally and physically aggressive than were their French counterparts. The American teens also spent less time leaning against, stroking, kissing, and hugging their peers. A similar study compared touching behavior in preschool children at playgrounds and in McDonald's restaurants in Paris, France, and in Miami, Florida.[27] The Parisian preschoolers touched each other more, were touched more often by their mothers, and were less aggressive toward their peers than were the American preschoolers.

Anthropologist J.W. Prescott has conducted research on the relationship between violence in society and positive touch interactions.[28] His findings reveal that the less physical affection received by children in a society, the greater the amount of violence among adults in that society. Prescott's theory, which is based on his research in 49 societies, suggests that children deprived of physical affection in childhood seek sensory experiences (drug use, delinquent behavior, crime as adults) to compensate for that loss of contact.[29]

A colleague recently related her experience with friends from Saudi Arabia, whose social speaking distance was much closer than that deemed comfortable by most Americans. It was easy to tell from afar, she said, which of 2 people involved in a discussion was from the United States. The American would retreat by inches from the Saudi, who then obligingly stepped forward to close the social distance as they slowly moved around the room. She mentioned that men in some areas of the Arab world hold hands or kiss each other in greeting, as do many Middle Eastern women. "Once I was seated on a sofa between my Saudi friends Nadia and Amira," she said. "We were involved in our discussion, and we were sitting very close together. I realized that as we talked, Nadia had been running her fingers lightly through my hair in a gentle caress. It was the most natural expression of friendship and affection, and I enjoyed her touch. Although her gesture was nonsexual, it would have been interpreted very differently by most Americans who observed it."

Maternal Touch
From my observations as a family physician, American mothers frequently touch their infants and young toddlers, but maternal touching decreases in frequency or may be disapproved of as children age. The blending of families may contribute to fewer instances of touching between parents and children in our society; for example, step-parents may hesitate to touch their stepchildren to avoid being misunderstood.

Studies demonstrate that positive touch is extremely important to development in infants.[30,31] Several decades ago, when neonatal medicine emerged as a medical specialty and physicians became more successful in resuscitating premature infants, many newborns in the United States were isolated in neonatal intensive care units (NICUs). They were sustained by tube feedings, supplemental oxygen, and intravenously administered medications and fluids. Because of concern about maintaining oxygen levels and the possible displacement of tubing, these babies were touched infrequently. Realizing the long-term effects of touch deprivation, a group of NICU nurses led research interventions to study the effects of touch stimulation in premature infants.[32,33] Their research confirmed that touching those babies caused no harm and improved their growth and development.

Many mothers have taken their newborn baby to the hospital for required blood tests. One study measured the effects of heelsticks in infants who were held by their mother during the procedure and in infants placed in a crib and separated from their mother during the blood draw.[34] A significant decrease in pain (an 82% reduction in crying and a 65% reduction in grimacing) was noted in babies who were held by their mother during the procedure. The researchers concluded that the skin-to-skin contact between a mother and her newborn was a potent pain reliever. Many physicians, however, are taught to take a child or infant to an isolated room away from the parent if performing a painful procedure is necessary.

Other research indicates that skin-to-skin contact between a mother and her infant promotes bonding. In one study, premature babies who had been caressed and positively touched by their mother exhibited good social and emotional health at 2 years of age.[35] The premature infants of mothers who provided much less nurturing and more negative touch interactions (pinching, slapping) showed signs of anxiety and social withdrawal at 2 years of age. The type of touch interaction was a more accurate indicator of a child's psychosocial development than were maternal displays of emotional warmth or other facets of child care.[36]

The frequent use of daycare facilities for American infants, toddlers, and preschoolers and the competitive environment of those facilities further reduces the opportunity for positive touch. The Touch Research Institute in Miami, Florida, conducted a study on the frequency of such touching among staff and children in a model childcare facility in Miami. The study results showed that childcare workers touched 1-year-old children less than 12% of the total day or shift spent in child care.[37] Other research indicates that touch deprivation in early childhood is associated with violent behavior in adolescence.[38] Infants in a nonaggressive and relatively peaceful culture like that of the !Kung people of the Kalahari Desert, however, have almost constant physical contact with their mother.[39]

In the past, children who received little positive touch at home might have received some affection (hugs, hand holding or squeezing, a light touch on the cheek or head to soothe emotions or offer comfort) from their schoolteachers. In America today, this occurs infrequently because many schools prohibit or discourage physical contact between students and teachers. Because touching may be misinterpreted as assault or molestation, it is discouraged even among members of blended families, hospitalized patients and their caregivers, and participants in activities sponsored by religious institutions such as church groups. Certainly an awareness of abuse is essential to societal health, but that fear must be balanced with a knowledge of the benefits that appropriate healing touch provides.

In the 1940s, scientific investigation of the effect of touch and social interaction in children was published in a clinical research project on nutrition in Germany.[40] Else Widdowson, a British dietitian, had been assigned to provide dietary supervision for 2 orphanages in Germany that provided care for children ranging in age from 5 to 14 years. Widdowson designed an experiment in which children at one of those orphanages received a significant increase in the daily rations of bread, orange juice, and jam. Children at the other orphanage received standard portions of those foods. Widdowson noted the weight and height of each child when the study began and several months later at the study conclusion. She was shocked by the results. The children who had received standard portions exhibited greater gains in height and weight than did those who had received extra rations. An investigation revealed the reason for those paradoxic findings. The overseer of the orphanage that distributed the extra rations was a strict disciplinarian who used punishment and intimidation to control her charges. She often scolded, rebuked, and publicly humiliated children during meals. The overseer of the orphanage that distributed standard portions had a kind, loving, and warm demeanor. She was frequently affectionate with the children and treated them with respect and understanding. Widdowson concluded that the wisdom of the proverb "Better a dinner of herbs where love is, than a fatted ox with hate therewith." confirmed her findings.[40]

Healing Touch

The first stethoscope, which was invented in 1816 by Rene Laennec, MD, caused much debate among physicians.[41] Before that event, physicians assessed human heart function by placing their ear on the patient's chest. Some doctors initially opposed the use of the stethoscope because they objected to creating a distance between the physician and the patient during examination.[42] Sadly, many physicians today impose another type of distance between themselves and their patients. The emotional and physical interaction of doctor and patient, which creates a bond of trust and confidence, is often diminished to a few minutes' duration. I believe that our heritage as physicians emphasizes the value of the patient-physician bond, which is a key element in diagnosis and treatment. Many healthcare givers overemphasize technology and medical intervention at the expense of the emotional and physical needs of their patients. In 1999, Sr. Mary, a Medical Mission Sister at St. Elizabeth's Clinic in Tucson, Arizona, said it well: "We must not let professionalism spoil the milk of human kindness!"

Research indicates the value of touch therapy in patients of all ages and in those suffering from any of a variety of disorders. Touch reduces the frequency of migraines and the level of pain during treatment for burns.[43,44] It enhances alertness, relieves anxiety, improves pulmonary function in patients with asthma, and helps to resolve dermatitis and chronic low back pain.[45-49] Patients with cystic fibrosis, bulimia, spinal cord injury, or attention-deficit disorder with hyperactivity have also been shown to benefit from massage therapy.[50-53] Touch therapy has also been shown to improve responsiveness in autistic children.[54,55]

Touch During Crisis
Can you recall being comforted by the touch of another human being when you were in the midst of an emotional or physical crisis? The most intense physical pain that I have ever experienced occurred during the birth of my first child. My exhausted husband, who is also a physician, had been on call the night before and had worked for more than 36 hours without a break. He had collapsed on a couch near the delivery room. The pain from one contraction was so severe that I thought I would lose consciousness, but I didn't want to complain to anyone. I felt a certain pressure to be a good patient in the hos-

pital where my daughter was born because I admitted patients and delivered babies there.

During the next contraction, a nurse was at my bedside to make some adjustments, and she unintentionally rested her hand very lightly on my hip while doing so. The subsequent contraction was less painful; it seemed as if her light touch had neutralized the pain. I was skeptical but observant. The nurse returned a short time later, and I had the same experience: Her gentle touch again lessened the severe pain of childbirth. I have also observed the analgesic power of touch as a mother. As soon as I am able to connect with one of my children who has been hurt, her sobs lessen, her breathing and heart rate decrease, and her pain usually dissipates.

Touch and Sentics

Sentics is the technique of capturing emotion on paper. In one study, investigators attempted to use a device called a sentograph to record the graphic pattern of platonic love.[56] Research subjects were asked to place the middle finger of one hand on the finger rest of the sentograph and exert pressure in response to emotion. Two pressure transducers measured the vertical and horizontal components of the pressure applied. A sentogram, which is the pattern of the applied pressure captured on paper as a diagram, has been created to represent several emotions. The pattern for platonic love, which was formed by the application of light pressure, appeared as a sweeping line directed toward the subject's body. Despite the fact that the research subjects were from diverse cultures ranging from highly industrialized societies to remote tribes, a consistent pattern emerged for several emotions, including compassionate love.

Manfred Clynes, PhD, an acclaimed musician and scientist, produced sentograms created after exposure to the music of Mozart, Beethoven, and Bach. Dr. Clynes demonstrated a connection of sentic forms related to the works of those great composers, as well as to works of art such as the *Pieta* by Michelangelo and *The Epiphany* by Giotto. Dr. Clynes captured on paper the power of science, art, and music to evoke the emotions of compassion, love, and reverence.

I have often observed positive changes in a patient's mental or physical status that were induced by compassionate interactions with caregivers as well as by listening to music or experiencing art. Those abstract languages lift our spirits, engender hope and awe, and help us forget our physical and psychic pain.

Compassionate Touch

When I was a medical student in my early 20s, I provided care for a male patient who was about my age. He had a degenerative neuromuscular disease and resided in a nursing home, but he had been hospitalized for the treatment of a severe infection. I noted that no family members or visitors came to his bedside. He was pale, gaunt, and contorted, and he appeared much older than his chronologic age. His eyes, however, were bright and intelligent as they peered from the prison of a bedridden body punctured with multiple tubes.

This patient breathed with a gurgling sound, and suctioning procedures that prevented his choking on secretions were frequently required. He was unable to speak and communicated by using his fingers to count out numbers. A signboard near his bed supplied the letter equivalent for the number of fingers he displayed: "A" was represented by 1 outstretched finger, E was signaled by displaying 5 fingers, etc. Because his communicating a sentence required a long time, most people did not want to "talk" with this patient. The evening before he was to be transferred back to the nursing home, I attended him, and he motioned for me to get the signboard. Using his tremulous left hand, he counted out the numbers 11-9-19-19. At first, I thought that he was making a mistake with the numbers, but then I realized that he was requesting a kiss from me. What he wanted most amid the horrors of his daily existence was a connection to another human being: intentional, caring touch. In that moment, I felt great compassion for him, and I kissed him.

Soothing Touch

A 40-year-old man hospitalized for the treatment of advanced leukemia was placed in isolation.[57] His family members could not touch him and had to stand away from his bed while wearing masks and gowns during their visits. His nurse was permitted to touch him, but he said that "She hated to touch me, or at least it felt that way. Whatever she was doing, she did with as little physical contact as possible." Deprived of touch, this patient became very depressed. He said, "I wish I could have told [my nurse] how important touch was. I craved the feeling of flesh on flesh. I craved it! It wasn't a sexual thing; in my condition, that was the last thing on my mind. But I really felt I was losing my will to live without that touch. I mean, I still wanted to live, to get better, but the reason to keep struggling was slipping away from me. I needed the feeling of someone's skin on mine to help me find it again."

I believe that many people feel that patient's isolation and share his emotions. They want — and need — touch to be a part of their therapy and cure. Humans share the universal burden of suffering. The connection made by the simple act of touching someone who is experiencing pain or stress provides much-needed comfort and communicates caring.

Comforting Touch

I once cared for a patient who was severely mentally retarded, deaf, blind, and mute. His medical condition required the placement of a nasogastric tube, which was to be inserted through his nose and advanced into his stomach. When I must perform a painful procedure, I usually use visual tools, music, or conversation to provide distraction or comfort. Because of this patient's sensory deficits, those methods weren't effective. Before we began, his caregiver pulled a feather boa from her bag and said as she handed it to me, "Here, he likes this." The patient responded positively to the light touch of the feathers and seemed to better tolerate his discomfort. His sense of touch was very much alive, and we used that modality effectively during his subsequent care.

Touch Therapy for Patients

I have included massage therapists as part of my clinical practice staff in several professional settings and have observed the value of this type of therapy. While I was practicing obstetrics as a family medicine physician, I supported the teaching of infant massage to new mothers in a birthing center. I also receive massage therapy on a regular basis. Massage therapy has many benefits, but it is not accessible to many of my patients because of its cost, the required time commitment, or problems with transportation. Some patients hesitate to schedule regular massage therapy because they consider it self-indulgent.

Interacting with animals through touch also provides health benefits,[58,59] and I often suggest that certain patients acquire a pet. However, pet ownership may not be possible for some patients, and others cannot afford or are not receptive to massage therapy. After searching for a type of touch therapy suitable for patients on a fixed income, people with a hectic schedule, and those with very limited economic and social resources, I discovered a solution: Bio-Touch.

Bio-Touch Therapy

I was introduced to Bio-Touch several years ago when I was working in Tucson, Arizona, at the St. Elizabeth of Hungary Clinic. St. Elizabeth's is a healthcare facility dedicated to providing medical and dental care for the working poor (individuals without health insurance). Mary Schild, MMS, came to the clinic once or twice weekly to perform Bio-Touch on our patients. Although I had observed that some patients seemed to benefit from that therapy, I knew little about Bio-Touch. One morning, I had a terrible migraine — and a full patient schedule. Tylenol and ibuprofen had been ineffective, and I was really struggling with headache pain. Like many working mothers, I had had to cancel my last 2 appointments for a therapeutic massage because of family needs. I was regretting those cancellations, because regular massage therapy helped to control my headaches.

My first patient cancelled her appointment just as Sr. Mary appeared. When Sr. Mary heard that a small window of free time had appeared on my schedule, she said, "Why don't you let me do Bio-Touch?" Because I had not learned about touch therapy or energy therapy in my medical training, I was really skeptical of that treatment, but I was desperate because my headache had not resolved. I was also open to learning about Bio-Touch, which had benefitted some of my patients. Because I wanted to test the effectiveness of the technique, I told no one (not even Sr. Mary) about my severe headache, which dissipated seconds after the treatment began. Then and there I decided to learn more about this modality, and I also began to refer more of my patients to St. Elizabeth's to receive Bio-Touch.

Bio-Touch: Simple, Affordable Touch Therapy

Bio-Touch is not part of a religious belief system, and no meditation or special consciousness is required to perform or receive it. Performing Bio-Touch requires no magnets or other devices, and it is easy to teach and to learn. Even children can be taught to perform the procedure successfully. I have found that someone who has just learned the technique (which requires a 2-day training course) is just as effective as a practitioner who has been performing Bio-Touch for 10 years.

During Bio-Touch, the practitioner uses the index finger and middle fingers of both hands to lightly touch combinations of 17 sets of designated points on the patient's body. Each point is touched for 6 to 8 seconds. This simple, hands-on technique seems to enhance healing. There is no hierarchy among practitioners of Bio-Touch, and the training of lay people (including children) is highly encouraged. Bio-Touch practitioners are forbidden to create expectations for the results of therapy. They provide no counseling, medical advice, or lifestyle suggestions. As a scientist and physician, I agree completely with those prohibitions. I have observed the consumer fraud perpetuated by some complementary and alternative therapies, which are often loosely regulated by professional societies and standards. Unfortunately, many desperate patients are perfect targets for healthcare scams.

The Bio-Touch Pilot Study

In 2002, I received the approval to conduct the pilot research project on Bio-Touch, the results of which were presented at the National Conference of the American Association of Integrative Medicine in San Antonio, Texas, in 2003.[60] The study was to be conducted at the healthcare facility at which I served as medical director of women's health.

Our first step in the research project was to teach the Bio-Touch technique to the staff who would administer the therapy. The International Foundation of Bio-Magnetics in Tucson, Arizona, sent instructors to train 29 healthcare providers (nurses, physicians, physician assistants, physical therapists, nursing assistants, volunteers) in the procedure. In the pilot research project, we wanted to consider the patient's perception of stress and pain relief as well as his or her physical and emotional status. We realized that events viewed as very painful or stressful to one individual may be perceived as only mildly painful or stressful to another.

When the study began, we used a quality-of-life questionnaire to evaluate each patient's physical pain and functioning, general health, vitality, social functioning, emotional status, and mental health. We enrolled 75 patients in the first phase of the study. Of those subjects, 96% were women educated to the college level, and 24.6% were women of color. Many of the participants stated that they enrolled because they wanted help for chronic pain, they were experiencing the effects of a high level of stress, or they suffered from frequent infections related to emotional stress. In all subjects, Bio-Touch therapy was used in addition to the patient's usual treatment for the condition to be addressed.

Each subject completed the quality-of-life questionnaire when the study began, 8 weeks later, and 4 weeks after the last Bio-Touch session. In each session, the practitioner performed the technique as taught but did not provide counseling, medical advice, or comments about the patient's response to the session.

I hypothesized that each subject would experience a reduction in stress and pain after 8 weeks of once-weekly therapy. We were amazed to find that after 8 weeks, all patients who completed the questionnaire indicated an improvement in **each** area of the quality-of-life questionnaire. I am aware of no drug that can induce those types of concomitant changes. Four weeks after the last Bio-Touch session, the subjects reported a sustained improvement in physical pain, social functioning, vitality, general health, and mental health.

Because of the body-mind connection, it is not surprising that when physical pain is relieved, improvements in physical function, vitality, and general health also occur. One chronic pain sufferer who participated in the study had, in her words, "maxed out the conventional medical approach to pain." She had undergone several surgeries and had been treated by physicians who specialized in providing pain relief. In spite of those efforts, she required narcotic medication each day to relieve her pain. She was in the process of applying for medical disability and stated that she had enrolled in the study because she had no options left and had little to lose. To her surprise, her chronic pain resolved over the 8 weeks of Bio-Touch therapy, and she withdrew her application for disability payments. When I inquired about her recently, I was told that she had just built a chicken coop and a fence on her ranch.

Not all subjects had such a dramatic response to Bio-Touch, but at the study conclusion, the participants reported a decrease in pain and improved physical function. Some women also lost weight during the study, although they had not changed their diet or exercise level. Many subjects reported experiencing a feeling of calmness, well-being, and serenity after each session. Most noted a decrease in restless mood, irritability, and agitation while they participated in the study.

The duration of the effects of Bio-Touch varied among the subjects. Some reported that they felt better immediately after a Bio-Touch session and for several hours or days thereafter. Others stated that they noticed an improvement in their symptoms 24 to 48 hours after a Bio-Touch session. Some reported that the chronic pain they had suffered for years had resolved and had not recurred. The study participants made the following comments about treatment with Bio-Touch:

"My back pain was eased for 5 days after the first Bio-Touch session."

"I don't have as much back trouble, and my headaches are less severe since I started the research study."

"I am in less pain with each session."

"Stress and depression are nonexistent for me for 5 to 6 days after Bio-Touch."

"I haven't had a headache in the 5 weeks since the study started."

"My back pain was gone after the first treatment and stayed gone."

"The numbness in my arm was gone after the first treatment. I came to the first session not expecting any difference, but after 15 minutes I felt great. It was amazing."

"My arthritis is better."

"I feel very relaxed."

"I have a sense of well-being after Bio-Touch."

"I really need these sessions. I don't know how I'll get through the week without them."

"My knees feel better."

"Bio-Touch is very calming. I'm in almost a presleep state after the touching begins."

"I have an increased feeling of well-being that lasts for 3 days after each session."

"Bio-Touch helped relieve my menstrual cramps."

"I've had hardly any discomfort in my neck since the first treatment."

"My chronic abdominal pain has subsided."

"I feel much less stressed."

"I lost weight without changing my diet."

"I have more energy, a decreased appetite, and fewer food cravings."

"I've had no sinus attacks during the 8 weeks of treatment, although I previously had chronic sinus infections."

"I've not had a migraine since the study started."

"I have more energy, especially in the evening. The effect of each session lasts about 5 days."

"I have had less of a problem with binge eating."

"I have been able to manage stress better."

"Bio-Touch relieved my carpal tunnel symptoms."

"I don't want to stop Bio-Touch treatments."

Bio-Touch produced an improvement in the quality-of-life scores of each participant. I believe that this study also showed the potential benefit of weekly interaction with a compassionate individual who affirmed the patient's reaction to stress and pain. I also concluded that the skin-to-skin contact between the practitioner and the patient may have conferred physical and psychologic benefits like those obtained from manicures, pedicures, cosmetic applications, hair styling, and massages. The subjects' reactions to Bio-Touch therapy suggest that skin is more than protection against the external environment. It is the interface of the external environment with the inner world of thoughts and feelings. For that reason, some chronic skin conditions (herpes, psoriasis, shingles, urticaria) worsen as emotional stress increases.[61]

After reviewing the data compiled during the Bio-Touch pilot study, we reached the following conclusions:

Practitioners trained to perform Bio-Touch therapy were proficient immediately after receiving training.

Bio-Touch therapy was well-accepted by the subjects and caused no adverse effects.

No equipment or special room was required to produce favorable therapeutic results.

Treatment with Bio-Touch once weekly improved all aspects of the patients' quality of life as indicated on the completed questionnaire.

Research Project 2: Effects of Bio-Touch in Healthy Postmenopausal Women

Our pilot project findings demonstrated that Bio-Touch improved physical, emotional, and social health in a diverse group of women. We then decided to further investigate the physiologic effects of Bio-Touch in a group of healthy women who were similar in age, ethnicity, hormonal status, education level, and lifestyle.

Research shows that after menopause, women have an increased risk of cardiovascular disease and age-related disorders such as dementia, cancer, and infections. We therefore decided to investigate the effect of Bio-Touch, a nondrug therapy, on the cardiovascular, immune, and stress-response hormone systems in healthy postmenopausal women.

My staff and I recruited 18 healthy postmenopausal women (age range, 62 – 84 years). Throughout the long history of medical research in America, women of that age have often been excluded from clinical research studies, although more American women now live well into the eighth decade of life.[62] I greatly enjoyed meeting the study subjects, and I especially appreciated their willingness to participate in the less popular arm of the study (the touch-deprived group described below), which was essential to our purpose.

The study participants had no serious chronic illnesses and were not receiving treatment with hormones, blood-thinning medications, steroids, or cholesterol-lowering medications during the study. All but 2 had a college education. About half of the women lived alone, and the remaining subjects lived with a spouse, an adult child, or an elderly parent.

We assigned 9 of the 18 women (the Bio-Touch group) to receive a 20-minute Bio-Touch session once weekly for 4 weeks in our medical center. The remaining 9 women (the no-touch group) agreed to abstain from touch interaction including massage, manicures, pedicures, and touch therapies for the study duration.

In both groups, levels of blood-clotting factors, inflammatory factors, estradiol, progesterone, cortisol, dehydro-epiandrosterone sulfate (DHEAS), and testosterone, and immune factors were measured at the initiation of the study and every other week by blood or saliva analysis.

Bio-Touch and Immune Factors

Interleukin-12 (IL-12) is a protein critical to the function of the immune system. It helps the body to fight infections and also prevents the growth of tumors. We found that during the second study, the women who received Bio-Touch exhibited levels of IL-12 that were **significantly higher** than those in the subjects who received no touch.

Research confirms that IL-12 levels decrease as we age and when we are emotionally stressed.[63,64] For that reason, older people may be more susceptible to infection and tumors, and women caregivers of a chronically ill spouse may exhibit the effects of a low level of IL-12 (delayed wound healing, more frequent infections).[65,66] Other factors that lower the IL-12 level include extreme exercise, undergoing a major surgical procedure, or sustaining a traumatic injury or a major burn.[67-69]

A low level of IL-12 may also contribute to the progression of a host of diseases and conditions: infection with *Helicobacter pylori*, tuberculosis, the human immunodeficiency virus, or the common cold viruses; severe allergies; asthma; and implantation failure after in vitro fertilization.[68,70] IL-12 is also administered experimentally or in research studies as a treatment for various types of cancer because of its tumor-fighting effect. It works by destroying newly formed blood vessels and new cancer cells.[71] Researchers have shown in animal studies that IL-12 is especially effective in inhibiting the progression of a precancerous breast tumor to malignancy.[72]

Bio-Touch and Cortisol

Cortisol is the hormone that regulates the metabolism of proteins, fats, carbohydrates, sodium, and potassium. It is released from the adrenal glands as part of the normal physiologic response to stress, which is often disrupted in older individuals, people experiencing emotional or physical trauma, and those suffering from depression, posttraumatic stress syndrome, panic disorder, or the effects of abuse or trauma that occurred during child-hood. The disruption of the normal stress response can cause an abnormally high level of cortisol.[73-77]

A persistently elevated cortisol level has been linked to the development of dementia, osteoporosis, cardiovascular disease, type II diabetes, and an increased susceptibility to infection or cancer (including breast cancer). [67, 68,78-82]

Some studies suggest that older women are more vulner-able to the disruption of the normal stress response and the ensuing long-term effects of excess cortisol than are men of the same age.[74,75,83] In the second Bio-Touch research study, half of the women in each group exhibited a high cortisol level when the study began. Of those women, the subjects in the no-touch group showed no improvement in their cortisol level during the study, but the women in the Bio-Touch group exhibited **a decrease** in their cortisol level.

Women who serve in the multiple roles of home worker, spouse, caregiver, mother, daughter, and community volunteer often experience the persistent unresolved psychologic stress that elevates the level of cortisol. Unfortunately, many of those women are unable to change the circumstances or relationships that cause that chronic stress. My research in women's health has shown that 2 safe and effective therapies (bioidentical progesterone and Bio-Touch) benefit women suffering from stress-related increases in cortisol. In Chapter 6, I explain the use of those treatments in correcting hormone imbalances in women.

Bio-Touch and Gene Expression

Genes are the units of heredity that transmit traits individual to each person, plant, or animal from the previous generation. Composed of deoxyribonucleic acid (DNA), genes are carried on threadlike chromosomes in the nucleus of each cell. Humans have 23 pairs of chromosomes, and each parent contributes 1 chromosome to every pair.

Gene expression (the effect of a particular gene) directs the development and function of the human body and all other living entities. However, the expression of some genes can be altered by the environment or by various physiologic processes. Genes like those that code for gender, eye color, and hair texture are static (ie, fixed), but most genes can be altered. This is a benefit. Having a gene associated with a disease does not mandate that the disease will develop. Diet, environment, lifestyle, socioeconomic status, drug or tobacco use, and hormonal status influence the expression of genes. We do not have to passively wait for a particular type of gene expression and subsequent illness to occur. Positive intervention can be effective in some cases.

To better understand the effects of Bio-Touch on gene function, we obtained a skin biopsy before and immediately after a Bio-Touch session in a subgroup of postmenopausal women in the second study. Because of the expense of that type of investigation, we limited our gene study to 4 women who were similar in age, weight, ethnicity, and social status. We found that the Bio-Touch intervention produced a favorable effect by upregulating (ie, activating) genes important in immune system function; DNA repair; the response to wounding, pathogens, physiologic stress, and inflammation; communication among cells; and longevity (Figure). Genes shown to be

Figure. Effects of Bio-Touch on Aging and the Response to Stress*

IL-12, Interleukin-12.

*Source: Stephenson K, Neuenschwander P, Kurdowska A, et al, investigators. The Effects of Bio-Touch on Neuroactive Hormones and Inflammatory, Antithrombotic, Prothrombotic, and Immune Signaling Factors in Postmenopausal Women Study.

related to an increased risk of cancer and dementia were downregulated (ie, turned off). We did not measure the duration of those gene effects because our focus was on immediate changes.

Although our study was limited by the small number of subjects, the results suggest that in humans as in animals, skin-to-skin contact causes an immediate response of gene expression that may be important in promoting survival, and that even in older women, gene expression can be influenced by touch.

Bio-Touch and Social Bonding

The amount of social support that we receive, the frequency of our social interactions, and the quality of those interactions directly affect the function of the cardiovascular, endocrine, and immune systems.[84] Research links family relationships of poor quality or the loss of a parent during childhood to health problems that develop in adulthood: long-term increases in blood pressure, altered hormonal responses to stress, and an increased risk of cardiovascular disease and cancer.[85,86] Patients who have cancer, cardiovascular disease, or another chronic illness and who receive social support, have frequent social interactions, and feel cared for have a better quality of life and live longer than do similar patients without those benefits.[84]

How can physicians prescribe social interactions for isolated or highly stressed patients? Some of my widowed, divorced, or single female patients in poor health have few economic resources and are limited emotionally and physically by their illness. Many patients in those circumstances have told me that they have dissolved their friendships because they cannot reciprocate emotional and social support via telephone contact, providing birthday or holiday gifts, or attending social events. Bio-Touch sessions, however, offer a nonthreatening, easily accessible form of social interaction in which recipients are not required or expected to reciprocate emotionally, financially, or physically.

Bio-Touch and Aging

The rate at which we age may be related to our emotional stress level, diet, exercise, educational level, intellectual interests, socioeconomic status, and gender (Figure). Many current studies are examining the genes of healthy men and women 90 years of age or older to identify the genetic characteristics that enable good health during very old age.[87] One goal of this type of research is to develop antiaging medications for people who lack "longevity genes."

Because of improved living conditions and advances in medical technology, women today are living much longer than they did just a century ago.[88] Many women, however, do not experience an enjoyable quality of life because of accelerated aging that is increased by stress. Bio-Touch may protect against some negative effects of aging by enhancing endocrine and immune function in healthy postmenopausal women without increasing the levels of sex hormones, clotting factors, or inflammatory factors. It also exerts a favorable effect on cortisol levels and gene expression.

I am currently conducting research in 2 areas: the role of Bio-Touch in reducing emotional stress in working women and the effects of Bio-Touch on age- and stress-related disruptions of the immune system and hormone levels in both men and women. I have also been invited to present my latest research findings on Bio-Touch at the national conference of the American Association of Integrative Medicine in October 2004. It is my hope that more clinicians will investigate the use of Bio-Touch to enhance the quality of life and improve the health of patients of all ages.

Case Reports: Practical Applications of Bio-Touch

Case 1. The Friend in Need

The mother of one of my daughter's friends appeared to be in pain when I stopped at her home to drop off her daughter. This woman described severe pain in her rib area but had not experienced a fall or injury. She was waiting for her doctor to call her about an appointment time. Because of her distress, I offered to perform Bio-Touch while she was waiting for the call about her appointment, and she agreed. The Bio-Touch session required about 10 minutes, and my daughter and I then left for our home. The next afternoon, the mother came to my house looking refreshed and comfortable. I asked her how she was feeling, and she looked at me suspiciously and said, "I don't know what you did, but after you left, my pain was eased and I went to sleep. When I woke up this morning, it was gone, so I cancelled my appointment with my physician. What *is* Bio-Touch?"

Case 2. The Hurting Child

One of my daughters ran into the house and screamed that she had been bitten on her back by fire ants. I raised her shirt and immediately saw 2 large red welts on her back. I instructed her to remain still while I hurried to get ice and pain-relieving medication. She stopped me and said, "No, Mom, just do Bio-Touch. I don't want to take a pill or have ice on my back." With extreme skepticism, I agreed. I knew that performing Bio-Touch for that condition would not be harmful, but I doubted that it would help. Several minutes after I began the procedure, my daughter stopped crying, sat up suddenly, and asked to go outside to play. Her pain had resolved.

Case 3. Tailgate Healing

Frank Schuster, CP, brings the benefits of Bio-Touch to the poor and homeless in Tucson, Arizona. An engineer by profession, Frank volunteers as a Bio-Touch practitioner for the Giving Tree Outreach Program, a nonprofit organization that provides food and other types of support for the disadvantaged of Tucson. In a recent article in the *Just Touch News*,[89] he described the outcome of a typical Bio-Touch session:

> The evening was dreary and dark with a light rain falling as I drove toward my destination: the outdoor feeding of the poor and homeless in a poor Tucson neighborhood ... I drove into the muddy lot and parked. Volunteers were serving a hot meal to 60 to 70 people. I got out of the truck and lowered the tailgate. To my amazement, two people got out of a car and came toward the truck. A woman got out of another car, took a wheelchair out of the trunk, helped another woman into it, and whisked her toward my truck. Four people were gathered around the tailgate wanting Bio-Touch ... Every Thursday evening I hand out flyers and wait for someone to come over to the tailgate, sit down, and receive Bio-Touch. They always come; usually a few and sometimes many. Several watch from a distance. Children are always curious and usually play around the truck. They want to be touched and sometimes seem more receptive to [Bio-Touch] than adults.
>
> One boy about 10 years old, whom I touched repeatedly upon his insistence, came over one evening and sat down for his Bio-Touch session. He often watched while I touched others. That day he had a puzzled look. "Do you touch people for your job?" I said, "No, this is what I do in my spare

time." "What job do you do?" he asked. "I'm an engineer," I replied. He thought for a moment and then said, "I know. You are a faith engineer. You give people hope." I was speechless. I finished [his Bio-Touch session] and gave him a big hug and a weak thank you ... I closed up the tailgate and drove home with tears in my eyes. What are these strange encounters and conversations? I only know that Bio-Touch is a movement way beyond my doing.

Conclusion

Bio-Touch research confirms that we as women need to include this simple yet powerful modality in the care of our families and of each other. My prescription pad is useful in times of illness, pain, or stress, and I do not fail to prescribe medications appropriately. However, I have used Bio-Touch alone or in addition to other medical therapies countless times in the care of my children, husband, extended family members, neighbors, and friends when they have needed help with pain or stress-related symptoms. I have found it very helpful for family members who want to comfort a loved one during times of crisis or illness.

Adults and children are comfortable receiving and performing Bio-Touch. It is a safe therapy. I have noted that even children like to perform Bio-Touch to help their mother, grandmother, pets, and friends. Weekly Bio-Touch sessions can also be included in a wellness or health maintenance program for people without health problems.

I have personally benefitted from Bio-Touch in the management of several chronic medical problems. I have used it as an alternative to taking medications or undergoing invasive interventions to treat pain. Because Bio-Touch causes no adverse effects, I believe that it can be used to complement any other medical therapy or psychotherapy. It can be performed easily in the home or in a medical clinic, a hospital, or a nursing home. No special equipment, music, or environment is required to perform the technique. I have often received or performed Bio-Touch therapy during ongoing conversations, in a tent, in a restaurant, in a hallway, and during myriad other distractions. It has been effective in many circumstances, and I highly recommend its use.

In summary, it can be said that Bio-Touch therapy does no harm but instead provides a source of positive touch, creates a social connection, and improves immune system function and the response to stress. Those benefits can help women sustain good health throughout all phases of life.

Acknowledgements

I would like to acknowledge the valuable assistance of Nancy Creech, research coordinator for the Bio-Touch research projects; Megan Black, BSN, who provided outstanding support; and Karin Sanders, who volunteered her time as a Bio-Touch practitioner. Further recognition is due to my coinvestigators who supported these projects: Anna Kurdowska, PhD; Pierre Neuenschwander, PhD; Barbara Pinson, MD; Douglas Stephenson, DO; Janet Seliga, BSN, MN; and David P. Holiday, PhD.

Others who generously contributed their time, resources, and expertise to this research project are: V. Morhenn, MD; D. Patel, PhD; C. Zambers, PhD; D. Zava, PhD; Greg and Kathy Fergueson; Drenda Johnston, LVN; Jane Boreman, RN; Kathy Hayden, LVN; D. Shafer, MD; J. Stocks, MD; Patti Harvey; Jesse Lewis, RN; Rene McCarty, PA; Anne DeWett, MN; Sheila Lowry; Sandra Lehman; and the study patients who participated in the Bio-Touch research projects.

Suggested Reading

Wilson JL. *Adrenal Fatigue: The 21st Century Stress Syndrome.* Petaluma, Calif: Smart Publications; 2001.Web site: www.adrenalfatigue.org

Internet Resources

www.justtouch.com — International Foundation of Bio-Magnetics, Tucson, Ariz. To obtain a complete history of Bio-Touch and information about classes and training or to learn more about a Bio-Touch practitioner in your area, visit the Web site or call 877-323-7951.

www.salivatest.com — ZRT Laboratory, 1815 NW 169th Place, Suite 5050, Beaverton, OR 97006. To learn more about the use of saliva testing to determine cortisol levels, visit the Web site or call 503-466-2445.

References

1. Older J. *Touching Is Healing.* New York, NY: Stein and Day;1982:86.

2. Tiwari M. In: *Ayurveda: A Life of Balance: The Complete Guide to Ayurvedic Nutrition & Body Types with Recipes.* Rochester, Vt: Healing Arts Press; 1995:1-30.

3. Godolphin FRB, ed. *Great Classical Myths.* New York, NY: Random House Inc.; 1964.

4. Champagne F, Meaney MJ. Like mother, like daughter: evidence for non-genomic transmission of parental behavior and stress responsivity. *Prog Brain Res.* 2001;133:287-302.

5. Caldji C, Tannenbaum B, Sharma S, Francis D, Plotsky PM, Meaney MJ. Maternal care during infancy regulates the development of neural systems mediating the expression of fearfulness in the rat. *Proc Natl Acad Sci U S A.* 1998;95(9):5335-5340.

6. Caldji C, Liu D, Meaney MJ. Maternal care alters the development of stress induced norepinephrine release in the PVNh. *Soc Neuro Sci Ab.* 1999;25(1):619.

7. Fleming AS, Vaccarino F, Leubke C. Amygdaloid inhibition of maternal behavior in the nulliparous female rat. *Physiol Behav.* 1980;25(5):731-743.

8. Fleming AS, O'Day DH, Kraemer GW. Neurobiology of mother-infant interactions: experience and central nervous system plasticity across development and generations. *Neurosci Biobehav Rev.* 1999;23(5):673-685.

9. Nishijo H, Uwano T, Tamura R, Ono T. Gustatory and multimodal neuronal responses in the amygdala during licking and discrimination of sensory stimuli in awake rats. *J Neurophysiol.* 1998;79(1):21-36.

10. van Wimersma Greidanus TB, Maigret C. Grooming behavior induced by substance P. *Eur J Pharmacol.* 1988;154(2):217-220.

11. Ferguson JN, Young LJ, Hearn EF, Matzuk MM, Insel TR, Winslow JT. Social amnesia in mice lacking the oxytocin gene. *Nat Genet.* 2000;25(3):284-288.

12. Francis D, Diorio J, Liu D, Meaney MJ. Nongenomic transmission across generations of maternal behavior and stress responses in the rat. *Science.* 1999;286(5442):1155-1158.

13. Swiergiel AH, Takahashi LK, Kalin NH. Attenuation of stress-induced behavior by antagonism of corticotrophin-releasing factor receptors in the central amygdala in the rat. *Brain Res.* 1993;623(2):229-234.

14. Tsuchiya T, Horii I. Epidermal cell proliferative activity assessed by proliferating cell nuclear antigen (PCNA) decreases following immobilization-induced stress in male Syrian hamsters. *Psychoneuroendocrinology.* 1996;21(1):111-117.

15. Tsuchiya T, Nakayama Y, Sato A. Somatic afferent regulation of plasma corticosterone in anesthetized rats. *Jpn J Physiol.* 1991;41(1):169-176.

16. Tsuchiya T, Nakayama Y, Sato A. Somatic afferent regulation of plasma luteinizing hormone and testosterone in anesthetized rats. *Jpn J Physiol.* 1992;42(4):539-547.

17. Blalock JE. The syntax of immune-neuroendocrine communication. *Immunol Today.* 1994;15(11):504-511.

18. Young LJ, Winslow JT, Nilsen R, Insel TR. Species differences in V1a receptor gene expression in monogamous and nonmonogamous voles: behavioral consequences. *Behav Neurosci.* 1997;111(3):599-605.

19. Simonds PE. *The Social Primates.* New York, NY: Harper & Row; 1974:170-179.

20. Wang S, Bartolome JV, Schanberg SM. Neonatal deprivation of maternal touch may suppress ornithine decarboxylase via down-regulation of the proto-oncogenes c-myc and max. *J Neurosci.* 1996;16(2):836-842.

21. Bartolome JV, Wang S, Schanberg SM, Bartolome MB. Involvement of c-myc and max in CNS beta-endorphin modulation of hepatic ornithine decarboxylase responsiveness to insulin in rat pups. *Life Sci.* 1999;64(5):PL87-91.

22. Kuhn CM, Schanberg SM. Responses to maternal separation: mechanisms and mediators. *Int J Dev Neurosci.* 1998;16(3-4):261-270.

23. Goodall J. *In The Shadow of Man.* Rev. ed. Boston, Mass: Houghton Mifflin; 1988:244-246.

24. Hinde RA. Development of social behavior. In: Schrier AM, Stollwitz F, eds. *Behavior of Nonhuman Primates.* New York, NY: Academic Press; 1971:1-60.

25. Behrman RE, Kliegman RM, Nelson WE, Vaughn VC, eds. *Nelson Textbook of Pediatrics.* 14th ed. Philadelphia, Pa: WB Saunders

Company; 1992:13-21.

26. Field T. American adolescents touch each other less and are more aggressive toward their peers as compared with French adolescents. *Adolescence*. 1999;34(136):753-758.

27. Field TM. Preschoolers in America are touched less and are more aggressive than preschoolers in France. *Early Child Dev Care*. 1999;151:11-17.

28. Prescott JW. Affectional bonding for the prevention of violent behaviors: neurobiological, psychological and religious/spiritual determination. In: Hertzberg LJ, Ostrum GF, Field JR, eds. *Violent Behavior*. Great Neck, NY: PMA Publishing; 1990:95-124.

29. Prescott JW. Early somatosensory deprivation as an ontogenetic process in the abnormal development of the brain and behavior. In: Goldsmith EI, Moor-Jankowski J, eds. *Medical Primatology*. New York, NY: S. Karger; 1971:1-20.

30. Powell GF, Brasel JA, Raiti S, Blizzard, RM. Emotional deprivation and growth retardation simulating idiopathic hypopituitarism. II. Endocrinologic evaluation of the syndrome. *N Engl J Med*. 1967; 276(23):1279-1283.

31. Ottenbacher KJ, Muller L, Brandt D, Heintzelman A, Hojem P, Sharpe P. The effectiveness of tactile stimulation as a form of early intervention: a quantitative evaluation. *J Dev Behav Pediatr*. 1987;8(2):68-76.

32. Field T. Supplemental stimulation of preterm neonates. *Early Hum Dev*. 1980;4(3):301-314.

33. Field TM, Schanberg SM, Scafidi F, et al. Tactile/kinesthetic stimulation effects on preterm neonates. *Pediatrics*. 1986;77(5):654-658.

34. Gray L, Watt L, Blass EM. Skin-to-skin contact is analgesic in healthy newborns. *Pediatrics*. 2000;105(1):e14.

35. Feldman R, Weller A, Sirota L, Eidelman AI. Testing a family intervention hypothesis: the contribution of mother-infant skin-to-skin contact (kangaroo care) to family interaction, proximity, and touch. *J Fam Psychol*. 2003;17(1):94-107.

36. Moms' touch give kids social push. [feature]. *Science News*. 2001;160(18):280.

37. Field TM, Harding J, Soliday B, Lasko D. Gonzalez N. Valdeon C. Touching in infant toddler and preschool nurseries. *Early Child Dev Care*. 1994;98:113-120.

38. Field TM. Violence and touch deprivation in adolescents. *Adolescence*. 2002;37(148):735-749.

39. Konner MJ. Maternal care, infant behavior and development among the !Kung. In: Lee RB, DeVore I, eds. *Kalahari Hunter-Gatherers: Studies of the !Kung San and Their Neighbors*. Cambridge, Mass: Harvard University Press; 1976:218-245.

❖

40. Widdowson EM. Mental contentment and physical growth. *Lancet*. 1951;1(24):1316-1318.

41. 3M. History of stethoscopes. Available at: www.3m.com/us/healthcare/professionals/littmann/jhtml/history_of_scopes.jhtml. Accessed: August 12, 2004.

42. Fugh-Berman A. Why you should touch your patients. *Med Econ*. 1993;70(23):91-92, 94.

43. Hernandez-Reif M, Field TM, Dieter J, Swerdlow B, Diego M. Migraine headaches are reduced by massage therapy. *Int J Neurosci*. 1998;96:1-11.

44. Hernandez-Reif M, Field T, Largie S, et al. Children's distress during burn treatment is reduced by massage therapy. *J Burn Care Rehabil*. 2001;22(2):191-195; discussion 190.

45. Field T, Ironson G. Scafidi F, et al. Massage therapy reduces anxiety and enhances EEG pattern of alertness and math computations. *Int J Neurosci*. 1996;86(3-4):197-205.

46. Field T, Morrow C, Valdeon C, Larson S, Kuhn C, Schanberg S. Massage reduces anxiety in child and adolescent psychiatric patients. *J Am Acad Child Adolesc Psychiatry*. 1992;31(1):125-131.

47. Field T, Henteleff T, Hernandez-Reif M, et al. Children with asthma have improved pulmonary functions after massage therapy. *J Pediatr*. 1998;132(5): 854-858.

48. Schachner L, Field T, Hernandez-Reif M, Duarte AM, Krasnegor J. Atopic dermatitis symptoms decreased in children following massage therapy. *Pediatr Dermatol*. 1998;15(5):390-395.

49. Hernandez-Reif M, Field T, Krasnegor J, Theakston H. Lower back pain is reduced and range of motion increased after massage therapy. *Int J Neurosci*. 2001;106(3,4):131-145.

50. Hernandez-Reif M, Field T, Krasnegor J, Martinez E, Schwartzman M, Mavinda K. Children with cystic fibrosis benefit from massage therapy. *J Pediatr Psychol*. 1999;24(2):175-181.

51. Field T, Schanberg S, Kuhn C, et al. Bulimic adolescents benefit from massage therapy *Adolescence*. 1998;33(131):555-563.

52. Diego MA, Field T, Hernandez-Reif M, et al. Spinal cord patients benefit from massage therapy. *Int J Neurosci*. 2002;112(2):133-142.

53. Khilnani S, Field T, Hernandez-Reif M, Schanberg S. Massage therapy improves mood and behavior of students with attention deficit/hyperactivity disorder. *Adolescence*. 2003;38(152):623-638.

54. Escalona A, Field T, Singer-Strunck R, Cullen C, Hartshorn K. Brief report: improvements in the behavior of children with autism following massage therapy. *J Autism Dev. Disorders*. 2001;31(5):513-516.

55. Field T, Lasko D, Mundy P, et al. Brief report: autistic children's attentiveness and responsivity improve after touch therapy. *J Autism Dev Disord.* 1997;27(3):333-338.

56. Clynes M. *Sentics: The Touch of Emotions.* Garden City, NY: Doubleday/Anchor Press; 1977:16-51.

57. Parachin VM. The healing power of touch: the simple act of touching frequently reduces everyday anxiety and tension. *American Fitness.* 1991;9(6):40-43.

58. Jorgenson J. Therapeutic use of companion animals in health care. *Image J Nurs Sch.* 1997;29(3):249-254.

59. Edney AT. Companion animals and human health: an overview. *J R Soc Med.* 1995; 88(12):704-708.

60. Stephenson K, Pinson B, Seliga J, Black M, Holiday D. The effects of Bio-Touch on quality of life scores in patients. *Ann Am Psychother Assoc.* 2003;6(2):28.

61. O'Sullivan RL, Lipper G, Lerner EA. The neuro-immuno-cutaneous-endocrine network: relationship of mind and skin. *Arch Dermatol.* 1998;134(11):1431-1435.

62. Office of Research for Women's Health. National Institutes of Health Web site. Available at: www4.od.nih.gov/orwh/. Accessed June 24, 2004.

63. Douziech N, Seres I, Larbi A, et al. Modulation of human lymphocyte proliferative response with aging. *Exp Gerontol.* 2002;37(2-3):369-387.

64. Pawelec G, Hirokawa K, Fulop T. Altered T cell signaling in ageing. *Mech Ageing Dev.* 2001;122(14):1613-1637.

65. Glaser R, MacCallum RC, Laskowski BF, Malarkey WB, Sheridan JF, Kiecolt-Glaser JK. Evidence for a shift in the Th-1 to Th-2 cytokine response associated with chronic stress and aging. *J Gerontol A Biol Sci Med Sci.* 2001;56(8):M477-M482.

66. Kiecolt-Glaser JK, Marucha PT, Malarkey WB, Mercado AM, Glaser R. Slowing of wound healing by psychological stress. *Lancet.* 1995;346(8984):1194-1196.

67. Matalka KZ. Neuroendocrine and cytokines-induced responses to minutes, hours, and days of mental stress. *Neuroendocrinol Lett.* 2003;24(5):283-292.

68. Elenkov IJ, Chrousos GP. Stress, cytokine patterns and susceptibility to disease. *Baillieres Best Pract Res Clin Endocrinol Metab.* 1999;13(4):583-595.

69. Elenkov IJ, Chrousos GP, Wilder RL. Neuroendocrine regulation of IL-12 and TNF-alpha/IL-10 balance. Clinical implications. *Ann N Y Acad Sci.* 2000;917:94-105.

70. Ledee-Bataille N, Dubanchet S, Coulomb-L'hermine A, Durand-Gasselin I, Frydman R, Chaouat G. A new role for natural killer

cells, interleukin (IL)-12 and IL-18 in repeated implantation failure after in vitro fertilization. *Fertil Steril.* 2004;81(1):59-65.

71. Colombo MP, Trinchieri G. Interleukin-12 in anti-tumor immunity and immunotherapy. *Cytokine Growth Factor Rev.* 2002;13(2):155-168.

72. Gavallo F, Carlo ED, Quaglin E, et al. Prevention by delay: nonspecific immunity elicited by IL-12 hinders Her-2/neu mammary carcinogenesis in transgenic mice. *J Biol Regul Homeost Agents.* 2001;15(4):351-358.

73. Stones A, Groome D, Perry D, Hucklebridge F, Evans P. The effect of stress on salivary cortisol in panic disorder patients. *J Affect Disord.* 1999;52(1-3):197-201.

74. Wilkinson CW, Petrie EC, Murray SR, Colasurdo EA, Raskind MA, Peskind ER. Human glucocorticoid feedback inhibition is reduced in older individuals: evening study. *J Clin Endocrinol Metab.* 2001;86(2):545-550.

75. Hawkley LC, Burleson MH, Poehlmann KM, Berntson GG, Malarkey WB, Cacioppo JT. Cardiovascular and endocrine reactivity in older females: intertask consistency. *Psychophysiology.* 2001;38(6):863-872.

76. Heim C, Newport DJ, Wagner D, Wilcox MM, Miller AH, Nemeroff CB. The role of early adverse experience and adulthood stress in the prediction of neuroendocrine stress reactivity in women: a multiple regression analysis. *Depress Anxiety.* 2002;15(3):117-125.

77. Weber-Hamann B, Hentschel F, Kniest A, et al. Hypercortisolemic depression is associated with increased intra-abdominal fat. *Psychosom Med.* 2002;64(2):274-277.

78. Ferrari E, Cravello L, Muzzoni B, et al. Age-related changes of the hypothalamic-pituitary-adrenal axis: pathophysiological correlates. *Eur J Endocrinol.* 2001;144(4):319-329.

79. Polleri A, Gianelli MV, Murialdo G. Dementia: a neuroendocrine perspective. *J Endocrinol Invest.* 2002;25(1):73-83.

80. Black PH, Garbutt LD. Stress, inflammation and cardiovascular disease. *J Psychosom Res.* 2002;52(1):1-23.

81. Elenkov IJ, Webster EL, Torpy DJ, Chrousos GP. Stress, corticotropin-releasing hormone, glucocorticoids, and the immune/inflammatory response: acute and chronic effects. *Ann N Y Acad Sci.* 1999;876:1-11; discussion 11-13.

82. Elenkov IJ. Systemic stress-induced Th2 shift and its clinical implications. *Int Rev Neurobiol.* 2002;52:163-186.

83. Seeman TE, Singer B, Wilkinson CW, McEwen B. Gender differences in age-related changes in HPA axis reactivity. *Psychoneuroendocrinology.* 2001;26(3):225-240.

84. Uchino BN, Cacioppo JT, Keicolt-Glaser JK. The relationship between social support and physiological processes: a review with

emphasis on underlying mechanisms and implications for health. *Psychol Bull.* 1996;119(3):488-531.

85. Luecken LJ. Childhood attachment and loss experiences affect adult cardiovascular and cortisol function. *Psychosom Med.* 1998;60(6):765-772.

86. Russek LG, Schwartz GE. Feelings of parental caring predict health status in midlife: a 35-year follow-up of the Harvard Mastery of Stress Study. *J Behav Med.* 1997;20(1):1-13.

87. Abbott A. Ageing: growing old gracefully. *Nature.* 2004;428(6979):116-118.

88. Arias E. United States Life Tables, 2001. *Natl Vital Stat Rep.* 2004;52(14):1-38. Also available at: www.cdc.gov/nchs/data/nvsr/nvsr52/nvsr52_14.pdf. Accessed June 22, 2004.

89. Schuster F. Tailgate healing. *Just Touch News.* 2004;spring:6.

Appendices

It is important to remember that as women, we have many choices in all phases of life. The voice of Athena, the advocate of wisdom and illumination, resonates within us all. By listening to that intuition and discovering inner sources of hope and courage, we may — at any age and in any circumstance — make the choices that are best for ourselves and for those we love.

Appendices A, B, and C present the physical and emotional challenges faced by girls and women who have been my patients. It is my hope that readers will find helpful information in those profiles to discuss with their physician or healthcare professional. Because every woman's needs are unique, the case reports are not meant to substitute for diagnosis, clinical advice, or treatment. It is important not to change current treatment without first discussing that decision with a physician or other qualified healthcare provider.

Appendix A:
Case Reports — Girls, Adolescents, and Young Adults

Greek mythology tells us that Athena's mother, Metis, was swallowed by Zeus, Athena's father, to prevent the birth of their child. According to prophecy, a male child born of that union would be more powerful than Zeus himself. Held prisoner within Zeus, Metis worked diligently to fashion armor and a helmet that would protect Athena against evil. Her loud hammering caused Zeus to have headaches so terrible that he asked Hephaestus, the Greek god of fire and metalworking, for relief. Hephaestus split the head of Zeus with an ax, and Athena sprang forth, fully grown, fully armed, and brandishing a shield. Thereafter she was known as the goddess of wisdom and war, among many other favorable attributes.

Like Athena, girls and young women in modern America must arm themselves with resilience to overcome trauma, disappointment, betrayal, and loss. The protection created by a loving caregiver, the power of an education, the cultivation of self-esteem, and the devotion to truth are attributes that sustain our daughters through the journey of childhood, adolescence, and young adulthood. This chapter is dedicated to my own daughters and to my nieces, who now range in age from 8 to 26 years. I urge them to listen to the wisdom of their elders and to arm themselves with education and truth, because those weapons of defense can never be taken away. I counsel them to protect and defend their dignity and worth. Their generation has untold opportunities brought forth by advocates and activists who fought selflessly to ensure the freedom and equality of women in this country. Perhaps young women today will see the glass ceiling shattered, and their accomplishments and achievements will reach even greater heights.

The case reports in this Appendix, which I have recorded during years of clinical practice, address medical problems often experienced by girls and women in the first phase of the feminine life cycle (from birth to 30 years). I hope that the solutions presented here will be helpful to readers searching for similar answers, but each patient's medical and emotional needs are unique. It is important to remember that current treatment should not be changed without consulting a physician or healthcare professional.

Case 1. Overweight and Unhappy

AA, a 7-year-old girl, was brought to our office by her mother for the treatment of obesity. At the age of 2 years, AA was at the upper limit on the weight growth chart for children, and her weight had increased disproportionately to her height since that time. AA stated that she wanted to lose weight, and her mother was concerned about the effects of childhood obesity.

AA was a good student in the first grade of a public school. She ate breakfast and lunch in the school cafeteria as part of the school lunch program. After school she attended a daycare program from which her mother picked her up in the evening. AA and her mother usually ate fast food on the way home.

AA stated that she had no close friends in the neighborhood or at school. She spent evenings and weekends watching television or playing computer games. She did not participate in sports or exercise. Her mother mentioned that their neighborhood was not safe for bike riding, walking, or skating and said that she did not want to deny her daughter food, which was one of AA's few pleasures.

At the time of her examination, AA was being treated with no medications. She reported no prior major illnesses and had undergone no surgeries. She had not yet begun to menstruate. AA's mother was overweight and suffered from chronic migraines, and her father's health status was unknown. Both maternal grandparents suffered from high blood pressure and were obese and diabetic. The results of physical examination confirmed that AA was obese and that her blood pressure was slightly elevated. Her laboratory tests were within normal ranges.

Diagnosis
Childhood obesity

☞ *Treatment*
I recommended that AA's mother not base punishment or praise on her daughter's weight or food consumption. I also suggested AA should:

- Eat breakfast at home, take a nutritious lunch to school, and reduce her fast-food intake.

- Eat 3 evening meals at home with her mother each week. Children who often eat at home exhibit improved academic performance and behavior, better peer relationships, and improved self-esteem.[1]

- Participate in grocery shopping and meal preparation.

- Choose skim milk and water to drink with meals eaten at home and with a packed lunch.

- Avoid purchasing sugar-containing soda, candy, and ice cream for daily consumption at home.

- Start an exercise program with her mother. Although exercising outside in AA's neighborhood was not safe, she and her mother could easily enjoy a variety of indoor physical activities together: exercising to workout videos obtained from the local library, jumping rope, or dancing. Walking expends 325 calories per hour; dancing, 395 calories per hour; and aerobic exercise, 505 calories per hour.

- Join her mother in wearing a pedometer to monitor daily exercise.

- Enroll with her mother in a community recreation program.

- Practice yoga for kids 1 to 3 times weekly (see Chapter 3).

- Reduce the amount of television viewing and computer time to 2 hours or less per day. When I was discussing media goals, AA's mother commented with some frustration, "If she doesn't watch TV, what is she going to do?" AA quickly answered, "Mommy, I can do things with you!"

- Begin a handwork project with her mother. Hearth Song (www.hearthsong.com, telephone:

800-325-2502) is an excellent resource for hand-work projects that mothers and daughters can share. Magic Cabin (www.magiccabin.com, telephone: 888-623-6557) also offers high-quality natural products for craft projects that girls and women might enjoy (see Chapter 5).

- Undergo Bio-Touch sessions once weekly to reduce stress (see Chapter 7).

- Adopt a pet for AA, who would benefit from that companionship.

☞ Suggested reading

Spangel L. *Life is Hard, Food is Easy: The 5-Step Plan to Overcome Emotional Eating and Lose Weight on Any Diet.* Washington, DC; Lanham, Md: Lifeline Press; 2003.

Schlosser E. *Fast Food Nation: The Dark Side of the All-American Meal.* Boston, Mass: Houghton Mifflin; 2001.

Freymann S, Elffers J. *Dog Food.* 1st ed. New York, NY: Arthur A. Levine Books; 2002. — A guide to fun food creations made from fresh fruits and vegetables; popular with teachers and parents in my practice.

d'Avila-Latourrette V-A. *Twelve Months of Monastery Soups.* New York, NY: Broadway Books; 1998. — A cookbook of recipes for tasty soups made from seasonal fruits and vegetables.

☞ Cinematherapy for AA's mother
- *Super Size Me*

Follow Up

At AA's 8-week follow-up appointment, she and her mother had been able to make a few of the recommended changes; however, their exercise efforts had been thwarted by a lack of transportation to exercise class. AA was eating breakfast at home a few times per week and was taking her lunch to school. She and her mother were drinking more water and fewer sugared, carbonated beverages, and AA had lost 7 pounds.

Discussion

Research shows that rate of obesity in the US pediatric and adolescent population has doubled in the last 2 decades.[1] In the United States today, 15.3% of children 6 to 11 years of age and 15.5 % of those who are 12 to 19 years old are overweight or obese.[1] Multiple factors (greater consumption of high-fat or high-sugar foods, a lack of exercise, increased television viewing and computer game use, larger portions of food served in restaurants, greater emotional stress, demanding parental work schedules) are thought to contribute to that national trend. Children in lower socioeconomic groups are most at risk for obesity. A recent study demonstrated that obese children and adolescents have a health-related quality of life as low as that reported by children with cancer.[2] In every area measured (emotional, social, school functioning), the quality-of-life scores of obese children were lower than those of their normal-weight peers. The obese children were also absent from school more often than were their peers of normal weight.

Preventing and treating obesity require the dedicated efforts of physicians and healthcare providers, schools and teachers, parents, and the community. Some of my patients who are teachers or school nurses have initiated antiobesity projects in their schools. One teacher was concerned that some of her grade-school students drank only sugared sodas at breakfast, lunch, and dinner. She purchased a bottled-water dispensary for her classroom and found that the children enjoyed drinking cool spring water. Some of her students even made spring water their beverage of choice. Another school nurse designed a program for parents that provided information about pediatric health problems caused by childhood overweight and obesity and offered practical, affordable suggestions for prevention and intervention. From my clinical perspective, the most powerful force in helping obese children to lose weight is the support of a caring individual who models and promotes a healthful diet and lifestyle.

References

1. Krebs NF, Jacobson MS; American Academy of Pediatrics Committee on Nutrition. Prevention of pediatric overweight and obesity. *Pediatrics*. 2003;112(2):424-430.

2. Schwimmer JB, Burwinkle TM, Varni JW. Health-related quality of life of severely obese children and adolescents. *JAMA*. 2003;289(14):1813-1819.

Case 2. Afraid of the Sandman

BB, an 8-year-old girl, had difficulty falling asleep. Her mother requested a sleep-inducing medication for BB to ensure rest and to relieve anxiety at bedtime. BB lived with her parents and siblings (a brother and a sister). She attended second grade, was an excellent student, and exhibited normal social development. Both her parents worked full-time outside the home.

When I examined BB, she said that she could not fall asleep and that she was afraid to sleep. She denied having nightmares, difficulty at school, or problems with siblings or friends. Her mother noted that BB often became anxious and then agitated at bedtime. Attempts to calm her were ineffective, and she willingly went to bed only when she slept in her parents' bedroom, which was an unacceptable long-term solution. Treatment with diphenhydramine (Benadryl), acetaminophen plus diphenhydramine (Tylenol PM), and providing incentives for going willingly to bed were ineffective. The mother reported that her family had recently moved into a new home and that BB shared a room with her younger sister. She also mentioned that the family had moved 5 times in the last 7 years because of her husband's employment requirements. BB, however, said that she liked her new school and teacher. She had cable television in her room, and her parents did not monitor the programs that she watched or the number of hours that she spent viewing television.

At the time of her examination, BB was being treated with no medications. She had undergone no prior surgeries and had had no major illnesses. Her parents and siblings were healthy. Both of her grandmothers had suffered from phobias. An aunt who experienced anxiety attacks had been diagnosed as having bipolar disorder.

The results of BB's physical examination were in the normal range. No medical tests were deemed necessary.

Diagnosis
Sleep resistance

☞ Treatment
Instead of simply writing a prescription to relieve insomnia, I wanted to create a nonstressful interaction between BB and her parents that would provide a greater long-term benefit. BB's mother explained that she and her husband had recently experienced work-related pressure, a move to a new city, and financial worries in addition to the routine stress of parenting 3 children. They were becoming frustrated with the added emotional demands of BB's sleep resistance. I suggested, however, that BB's mother recognize the importance of her daughter's anxiety and that she encourage BB to express her thoughts and emotions rather than requiring her to be compliant and quiet. I suggested that the television be removed from BB's bedroom and that her parents monitor her television viewing. I thought that the prospect of sleep might be less frightening for BB if she were reassured by her parents' physical presence. Her mother or father could remain sitting in or near BB's bedroom while engaged in

handwork, reading, or another quiet activity until BB fell asleep. I also recommended the following therapy for BB:

- Avoiding caffeine. Often, parents do not realize that beverages such as carbonated sugared sodas or iced tea contain a dose of caffeine that can significantly affect a child.

- A Bio-Touch session performed by her mother each night at bedtime (see Chapter 7).

- Following a pleasant bedtime ritual, such as story reading or the use of "fairy dust" or having BB's mother bestow a dream wish with a "fairy wand."

- Sleeping on a special "dream pillow" filled with sleep-enhancing herbs (lavender, rosemary).

- Completing a handwork project (see Chapter 5).

- Practicing yoga 1 to 3 times weekly (see Chapter 3).

- Chronicling daydreams and night dreams in a journal.

☞ *Suggested reading for BB's mother*

Ban Breathnach S. *Romancing the Ordinary: A Year of Simple Splendor.* New York, NY: Simple Abundance Press/Scribner; 2002. — A source of dream pillow recipes.

Brown LM, Gilligan C. *Meeting at the Crossroads: Women's Psychology and Girls' Development.* New York, NY: Ballantine Books; 1993; and Cambridge, Mass: Harvard University Press; 1992.

Carey D, Large J. *Festivals, Family and Food.* Gloucestershire, United Kingdom: Hawthorne Press; 1986. — Ideas for creating celebrations and rituals that can impart a sense of security and a constancy of hearth and home.

☞ **Internet resource**
www.chinaberry.com — A source of fairy wands, fairy dust, and a variety of wholesome books for children. To request a catalog, call 800-776-2242.

Follow Up

After 1 month of having followed the recommendations listed above, BB reported feeling less anxious around bedtime. She said that on most evenings, she fell asleep without difficulty.

Discussion

Sleep resistance in childhood may be related to anxiety or fear. BB's medical history revealed that several members of her extended family suffered from psychiatric disorders and phobias thought to have a genetic basis. Research has shown that unsupervised television viewing may be related to sleep difficulties in children.[1] This may be due to images that engender fear or insecurity and to a child's inability to filter out negative images by rationalization. Studies indicate that teenagers and adults can rather easily dismiss negative images but that younger children may not have that capacity.[1] Children whose family history reveals members with anxiety disorders or who move frequently and thereby lose friends and change schools may be more vulnerable to the negative messages or images conveyed by television.[2]

Young children perceive the images seen on television as reality. They may fear that people or creatures featured onscreen will exit the television and arrive in their bedroom. In children, daily television viewing of more than 1 to 2 hours has been associated with an increased risk of learning and behavior disorders, academic difficulties, bulimia and anorexia, obesity, a belief in stereotypes, substance abuse, aggressive and violent behavior, and earlier sexual activity.[1] I recommend no television viewing by infants and toddlers. Research has shown that television viewing by that age group has been linked to the later development of learning and behavior disorders.[1] Instead of watching television, very young children should be playing, crawling, singing, and exploring. I recommend a limit of 1 hour of television viewing per day by children who range in age from 3 to 7 years and a 2-hour daily limit for children older than 7 years and adolescents. I strongly suggest that a television not be kept in the bedroom of children younger than 10 years of age. The temperament of older children and teenagers should also be considered before they are permitted to have a television in their room. I recommend that parents monitor the viewing habits of their children and teach the value of watching educational, informative, and nonviolent programs. Children who want to view a controversial program should do so with a parent or guardian. Such programs can encourage frank discussions about values, drugs, sex, violence, and stereotyping.

References

1. American Academy of Pediatrics. Committee on Public Education. American Academy of Pediatrics: Children, adolescents, and television. *Pediatrics.* 2001;107(2):423-426.

2. Healy JM. *Endangered Minds: Why Our Children Don't Think.* New York, NY: Simon and Schuster; 1990.

Case 3. Headaches, Stomachaches, and Heartaches

CC was a 10-year-old girl who complained of new-onset headaches and stomachaches. She had not noticed headache-associated changes in vision, hearing, speech, balance, or other brain functions and had not experienced weight loss, vomiting, or bowel changes related to the abdominal pain. However, her headaches and stomachaches caused her to visit the school nurse several times weekly, and she complained of both disorders at home. Her mother denied changes in CC's diet, home routine, or school activities. When she experienced a headache or stomachache, CC was effectively treated with Tylenol or Pepto Bismol or was encouraged to rest.

CC's medical history and the results of her physical examination were unremarkable. The only medications that she was taking were acetaminophen and Pepto Bismol as needed. When she was a toddler, CC had undergone the placement of tubes in both ears to prevent recurrent ear infections but had experienced no other surgeries. She had not yet begun to menstruate and had had no prior major illnesses. Her parents and siblings were healthy.

When I examined CC, she was in the fifth grade. She stated that she liked school and that she enjoyed playing on a soccer team and riding her bike. She had lived in the same neighborhood for 5 years and had friends in the neighborhood as well as at school.

During CC's physical examination, her mother left the room to check on her other children in the waiting room. I asked CC whether anything was bothering or worrying her that we had not yet talked about, and she became tearful. She said, "My grandfather died. I didn't get to say goodbye. My parents wouldn't let me go to the funeral. I don't want to talk about it to my Mom, because it will make her sad."

Diagnosis
Grief reaction

☞ Treatment
I referred CC to a local hospice that provided grief support for families and to the GriefNet Web site (www.griefnet.org), which has a special page designed for children. I encouraged CC and her mother to discuss

their feelings of sadness and loss with each other, with other family members, and with their minister. As treatment for CC's grief and sense of loss, I suggested that she write a letter to her grandfather in which she said good-bye to him and that she create a memory book or video about her grandfather. I also recommended that CC ask her grandmother if she could select an item (a book, photo, or pin) that had belonged to her grandfather and keep it in her room. In addition, I prescribed the following regimen:

- Treatment with Tylenol or Pepto Bismol in the dosage recommended on the product label as needed to treat headaches or stomachaches that recurred.

- Practicing yoga 1 to 3 times weekly (see Chapter 3).

- Completing a handwork project (see Chapter 5).

- Bio-Touch sessions when headache or stomachache occurred or at least once weekly (see Chapter 7).

☞ *Suggested reading for CC's mother*
Cobb N. In *Lieu of Flowers: A Conversation for the Living.* New York, NY: Pantheon Books; 2000.

Follow Up
At her 4-week follow-up visit, CC reported that she was experiencing fewer headaches and stomachaches at home and at school. She had maintained her grades and had begun to spend time with her friends and to engage in social activities. CC's parents had taken her to visit her grandfather's grave, and she was participating in a grief support group.

Discussion

Like adults, children experience sorrow and loss, but in our society their grief is often unrecognized and unacknowledged. We strive to shield children from discussions about death or to prevent their attending a funeral because we do not want to burden them with sadness. It is alarming for a child to see his or her parents cry or grieve, but death is a part of life, and we should appropriately reveal our feelings to our children. Grief is a normal response to a variety of losses such as the death of a loved one, divorce, or failing health. It may evoke a constellation of physical symptoms such as headaches, dizziness, palpitations, the feeling of a lump in the throat, nausea, decreased appetite, shortness of breath, tightness in the chest, fatigue, or difficulty sleeping.

Denial, anger, guilt, and acceptance are the recognized stages of grief. The duration of each stage varies with each experience, although intense physical symptoms usually subside 6 to 8 weeks after the event. In my clinical experience, sharing the grief caused by personal loss with a caring friend or family member is the most powerful factor in recovery. However, many families in our culture avoid talking about death or the deceased, as in the case of CC (who did not want to upset her mother by grieving) and CC's mother (who wanted to avoid exposing her daughter to the funeral of a loved one).

The death of a pet introduces many children to grief. It is important to eulogize the deceased pet, to create a memorial to its memory and bury it in a grave, and to allow tears. When my daughter was in first grade, her beloved dog died, and she expressed her feelings. "Mommy," she said, "my chest hurts. It feels like it is going to blow up, and I can't breathe right. I feel like my heart is broken because my only true friend has died." By letting our children see the mystery of death, participate in the pancultural experience of grief, and share their heartache, we honor them as human beings.

Case 4. A Child No More

DD, a 12-year-old girl, was brought to my office for the treatment of what her foster mother described as "female problems." DD was an only child without an extended family. The identity of her father was unknown; he rejected parenthood and had abandoned his pregnant partner before DD was born. Her mother, who had had a traumatic childhood and no social support during her pregnancy or postpartum period, was institutionalized long-term for the treatment of an undisclosed psychiatric illness when DD was about 3 years old. DD was subsequently placed in several different foster-care settings, and she communicated with her mother sporadically via letters or rare visits. She had no memory of her preschool years. At the time of her examination, she was living with foster parents.

When asked about the onset of her symptoms, DD said that she had recently gone to a friend's home after school. Several male and female students, who ranged in age from 11 to 16 years, were playing a game of Truth or Dare at the house. No adults were home, and DD joined the game. When she refused to tell the truth, she was forced to take the dare, which in this case was nonconsentual sex. In childlike terms and without emotion, she described having been raped by a 16-year-old male who was also playing the game.

When I examined DD, she was being treated with no medications. She had undergone no prior surgeries and had had no major illnesses. She had begun to menstruate when she was 10 years old, and she denied prior sexual abuse. The results of laboratory testing for pregnancy and sexually transmitted infections were negative. Her physical examination was otherwise unremarkable.

Diagnosis
Sexual trauma, attachment disorder

☞ *Treatment*
Without overemphasizing the terrible trauma that DD had endured, I affirmed her suffering and anger. I suggested that DD's foster parents supervise and monitor her activities after school and on weekends and also recommended the following treatment:

- Counseling with a psychotherapist to develop DD's emotional resilience and to help her process and move beyond the traumatic experience of rape.

- Participation in a martial arts program and in school sports.

- If possible, the adoption of a pet for companionship and to develop nurturing skills.

- Completing a handwork project (see Chapter 5).

- Practicing yoga for kids to develop self-awareness and body awareness (see Chapter 3).

- Scheduling a Bio-Touch session at least once weekly to provide a source of positive, appropriate, nonthreatening physical contact (see Chapter 7).

☞ *Cinematherapy*
- *The Wizard of Oz*

- *Secondhand Lions*

☞ Suggested reading for DD

Creech S. *Ruby Holler*. New York, NY: Joanna Cotler Books/Harper Collins Publishers; 2002.

DiCamillo K. *Because of Winn-Dixie*. Cambridge, Mass: Candlewick Press; 2000.

☞ Suggested reading for DD and her foster mother to share

Madaras L, Madaras A. *The What's Happening to My Body? Book for Girls: A Growing Up Guide for Parents and Daughters.* New York, NY: Newmarket Press; 2000.

Follow Up

DD did not return for follow up.

Discussion

DD suffered from an attachment disorder. In medical context, "attachment" refers to the bond between an adult and a child. In an ideal situation, the adult in such a relationship provides an environment of security and trust that is necessary for the child's physical and emotional development. A child develops self-esteem and feelings of self-worth from the perception that a parent or caregiver loves and protects her and will meet her needs over time. Children in relationships that lack those attributes feel unloved and insecure. Research shows that children who are abused or neglected, especially during their first 3 years of life, are at great risk for not forming healthful attachments to anyone.[1,2]

Children who enter foster care (more than 500,000 in the United States in 2000) and those who experience life with many different caregivers, frequent moves, or inadequate parenting are at high risk for attachment disorder.[2] Physical and emotional abuse have also been shown to affect the normal stress response and subsequent behavior in children.[3] Some children react to environmental stress by detaching and disengaging emotionally. Others exhibit hyperactivity, anxiety, mood swings, or impulsiveness or develop sleep problems.

Research shows that treatment for attachment disorders can be effective and that children who are loved and valued by least 1 adult can overcome the trauma of abuse and neglect. Living in an environment of positive emotional constancy and permanency helps children to develop a sense of well-being.[2]

References

1. Boris NW, Zeanah CH. Clinical disturbances of attachment in infancy and early childhood. *Curr Opin Pediatr.* 1998;10(4):365-368.

2. American Academy of Pediatrics. Committee on Early Childhood and Adoption and Dependent Care. Developmental issues for young children in foster care. *Pediatrics.* 2000;106(5):1145-1150.

3. Perry BD, Pollard R. Homeostasis, stress, trauma, and adaptation. A neurodevelopmental view of childhood trauma. *Child Adolesc Psychiatr Clin N Am.* 1998;7(1):33-51.

Case 5. Inner Conflict, Inner Pain

EE, a 14-year-old female patient, complained of sharp, intermittent abdominal pain of 2 years' duration. The pain occurred either above or below the navel and persisted from several minutes to as long as 1 hour. The onset of pain was not associated with emotional or physical stress, menstruation, bowel movements, the ingestion of certain foods, or symptoms of other disorders. Although she experienced the pain on a daily basis, it was rarely severe enough to cause her to withdraw from scheduled activities. She had been evaluated by several other physicians before her visit to our clinic, but no effective treatment had been identified. EE stated, however, that she noted relief if she lay down at the onset of pain.

EE lived with both biologic parents. She was in the eighth grade, liked school, and had good grades. She denied social, family, or school conflicts and had several close friends. She enjoyed crafts and volunteered in her church and community. EE usually ate meals, which included fruits and vegetables, at home. She consumed neither caffeine nor alcohol and did not use tobacco or illicit drugs. Her primary forms of exercise were cycling and hiking. Her parents and siblings were in good health.

EE was being treated with no medications when she sought my help. She had undergone no prior surgeries and had had no major illnesses. She had begun to menstruate when she was 12 years of age. Her periods occurred every 28 to 32 days, and her menstrual flow lasted 5 to 7 days. She was not sexually active.

EE was slightly underweight. During her physical examination, no abdominal tenderness or other abnormality was noted. The results of laboratory analyses, including a complete blood count, a basic metabolic panel (a blood chemistry panel), a stool test, urinalysis, and thyroid hormone values, were within the normal range. Radiographic evaluation (x-ray films) of her abdomen revealed no abnormality.

Diagnosis
Recurrent abdominal pain syndrome

☞ Treatment
Adolescent girls may be less likely than younger girls or adult women to articulate their feelings, especially those of conflict. Their emotional distress is often manifested physically as episodes of abdominal pain. I reassured EE that recurrent abdominal pain syndrome is not life-threatening and prescribed the following:

- Keeping a calendar documenting the date, time, location, and duration of episodes of her abdominal pain.

- Consuming an adequate amount of fiber.

- Attempt to identify foods that might trigger the onset of pain.

- Receiving Bio-Touch therapy to her upper and lower abdomen once weekly and also when her abdominal pain occurred (see Chapter 7).

☞ **Suggested reading for EE's mother**

Myss C. *Anatomy of the Spirit: The Seven Stages of Power and Healing.* New York, NY: Harmony Books; 1996. — A discussion of mind-body connections in illness.

Pipher M. *Reviving Ophelia: Saving the Selves of Adolescent Girls.* Reissue ed. New York, NY: Ballantine Books; 1995. — An excellent analysis of the challenges faced by teenage girls.

Follow Up

At her follow-up examination 3 months after the initiation of treatment, EE said that Bio-Touch therapy seemed to be the most beneficial treatment. After she began that therapy, her daily episodes of abdominal pain diminished in intensity until they occurred less than once per month.

Discussion

Chronic abdominal pain is a common complaint in childhood and adolescence. It may have any of several causes (ulcers, inflammatory bowel disease, constipation, food intolerance). Recurrent abdominal pain syndrome is characterized by chronic abdominal pain. The diagnosis of the syndrome is based on the patient's symptoms and having ruled out other causes of the abdominal pain. This type of abdominal pain is not life-threatening. It is common in girls 8 to 12 years of age and usually resolves within several years.[1]

Management of recurrent abdominal pain syndrome includes acknowledging that the patient's pain is real and reassuring her that extensive testing will not be necessary for diagnosis. Encouraging the patient to record episodes in a symptoms diary and maintaining good rapport as a physician with the patient and her family members is important to the success of treatment.

Reference

1. Lake AM. Chronic abdominal pain in childhood: diagnosis and management. *Am Fam Physician.* 1999;59(7):1823-1830.

Case 6. Seized By Anxiety

FF, a 14-year-old female patient, was admitted to the hospital for the treatment of frequent severe seizures that had begun several weeks before her hospitalization. The frequency and severity of the seizures had increased over the last few weeks. During her hospitalization, FF was treated with sufficient doses of antiseizure medications, but the seizures continued to recur. She had undergone no prior surgeries and had experienced no major illnesses. Her menstrual periods had begun when she was 12 years of age and recurred regularly each month. She was not sexually active. Her parents and siblings were healthy, and no seizure disorders had been diagnosed in her immediate or extended biologic family.

FF was a public school student in the eighth grade in an affluent neighborhood. She liked school and denied the use of alcohol, tobacco, or illicit drugs. She said that her circle of friends had changed recently, but she would not elaborate. She tearfully stated that her patients had just told her that they were divorcing. She reported that her parents fought frequently but had "gotten along better" since FF had become ill.

The results of brain imaging, physical examination, and laboratory analyses that included extensive testing were within the normal range. When FF underwent an electroencephalogram (EEG), she demonstrated movements characteristic of seizure, but the results of the EEG were within normal parameters.

Later during the day after our team had made formal rounds, I visited FF in her hospital room. I asked her whether anything in addition to her parents' impending divorce was troubling her. Initially, she seemed reluctant to engage in conversation, but she suddenly asked me (the only female member of the medical team) whether I had been a cheerleader. When I answered her affirmatively, she quietly stated that she had not "made cheerleader," and we talked for a while about cheerleading and the implications of not being selected. I inquired about the date of the tryouts, and it coincided with the onset of her seizures.

Diagnosis
Pseudoseizures (a stress-related pseudoneurologic syndrome)

☞ Treatment
Knowing the social and cultural context of this patient was essential to correct diagnosis and treatment. The peer pressure to be selected as a cheerleader is overwhelming for many young girls in FF's social group. Girls who do not succeed in that activity are often overcome by a sense of despair and failure. I acknowledged FF's perception of the magnitude of that trauma. I then recommended the following regimen:

- Consulting with a psychotherapist, whose perspective might be helpful for FF during her parents' divorce and her adjustment to the loss of previously meaningful peer interactions.

- Developing interests in activities other than cheerleading, such as yoga or handwork (see chapters 3 and 5).

- A modality such as Bio-Touch for stress reduction (see Chapter 7).

- Keeping a private journal in which she recorded her feelings.

☞ *Cinematherapy*
  - *Spellbound* (2002)

  - *Mean Girls*

  - *October Sky*

Follow Up
After FF had followed the recommended treatment for some time, her seizures gradually diminished. She was able to form new peer relationships and to set new goals. She found extended family members who, in addition to her siblings, provided needed support during her parents' separation and eventual divorce.

Discussion
For many of my Texas patients, cheerleading is a family tradition in which the participation of girls and young women is much emphasized. The training for cheerleading and the formation of cliques devoted to that activity may begin as early as first grade. One of my patients, a 6-year-old girl, stated that other girls in her class would not let her sit at their table because she did not participate in the after-school cheerleading program.

FF felt overwhelmed by self-blame and guilt because of her failure in cheerleading. Her despair was further magnified by the impending divorce of her parents. Even though witnessing their arguments was stressful for FF, dissolving the family unit was a frightening and unknown experience. Children of divorcing parents often feel either responsible for the breakup or inadequate because they cannot keep their parents together. In addition, FF revealed that that her episodes of seizure kept both parents, who then fought less, near her bedside.

FF's pseudoseizures were caused by emotional stress. In American culture, the physiologic effects of psychologic distress are imposing: One estimate indicates that 25% to 72% of US patients seek help from their physician for the treatment of stress-related physical complaints.[1]

Pseudoneurologic syndromes, which are brought on by stress, can mimic any disease and can produce paralysis, deafness, or blindness. Patients (often adolescent girls or young adult women) who suffer from a pseudoneurologic syndrome cannot consciously express anguish caused by emotional stress. Instead, they manifest that anguish as physical symptoms with nervous system involvement. Thorough medical investigation, however, reveals no identifiable cause for their symptoms. Carefully interviewing and examining the patient are essential to the accurate diagnosis of pseudoneurologic syndromes.

Pseudoseizures like those experienced by FF can occur or worsen in the presence of others. The seizures seldom result in serious injury, despite the risk of falling. Patients who suffer any type of pseudoneurologic disorder should never be scolded or ridiculed but rather treated with compassion, support, patience, and encouragement until they can resume their normal function.

Reference

1. Shaibani A, Sabbagh M. Pseudoneurologic syndromes: recognition and diagnosis. *Am Fam Physician.* 1998;57(10):2485-2494.

Case 7. Silenced By Authority

GG, a 15-year-old female patient, had been in my care for several years. GG was an only child. She attended an exclusive private boarding school in another state. I typically saw her 2 to 3 times each year for the treatment of minor health problems or to perform a physical examination required by her school. When GG was a toddler, her mother died. Subsequent child care was provided by her father and a nanny or housekeeper until she was sent away to boarding school at the age of about 8 years.

When GG was 15, she suddenly flew home at midsemester and requested an urgent appointment for the evaluation of headaches. During the interview that preceded GG's physical examination, she seemed distant and evasive when questioned about her symptoms. She then divulged that she had experienced no headaches but that at a school dance a few weeks before, she had been raped by a young man who attended an exclusive boys school located nearby. She had immediately called her father, who had firmly instructed her to "keep quiet and forget it" because the rapist's father was an important business client. GG pled with me not to tell her father that she had confided in me and begged me not to document the incident in any medical record that her father could access. She said that since the rape she had been unable to sleep and had experienced episodes of rapid heartbeat, decreased appetite, chest tightness, shortness of breath, and intrusive thoughts that interrupted her concentration. She felt overwhelmed by the feeling of powerlessness in her relationship with her father and furious at the lack of consequences for the perpetrator.

GG was an excellent student who did not smoke or drink alcohol. She participated actively in sports at the boarding school that she attended, and she had several close friends. GG's nanny had been the most influential adult female figure in her life. Her father was a prominent, affluent society figure. GG, dressed in elegant attire, often served as his escort.

At the time of her examination, GG was being treated with no medications. She had experienced no prior surgeries or major illnesses. Her menstrual periods, which occurred every 28 to 30 days, had begun when GG was 12 years old. The results of her physical examination were in the normal range, although she was anxious and tearful during her examination. Her physical development was appropriate for her age. The results of laboratory testing for pregnancy and sexually transmitted infections were negative. GG's father was healthy, and she did not know the health status of her grandparents.

Diagnosis
Sexual trauma, posttraumatic stress disorder

☞ Treatment
My acknowledgement of GG's feelings of betrayal, my validation of the emotional and physical pain that she had experienced, and my willingness to hear her story seemed to provide some comfort. Because of my concerns about both the short-term and long-term effects of the trauma of rape, I recommended the following therapies:

- Treatment with eye movement desensitization and reprocessing (EMDR), a therapy effective in the treatment of posttraumatic stress disorder.[1] During an EMDR session, the patient recalls a past or present traumatic experience in brief episodes while simultaneously performing a series of eye movements or focusing on an external stimulus such as auditory tones or tapping. That segment of therapy is followed by a rest period, after which the patient associates a positive thought with the unpleasant event.

EMDR therapy can eliminate or greatly decrease the emotional distress that is related to memories of traumatic events, even if they occurred years ago. According to one study, three 90-minute sessions of EMDR eliminated posttraumatic stress disorder in 90% of rape victims.[2] Other research showed that sessions of EMDR reduced psychologic distress scores in traumatized young women and brought those scores within 1 standard deviation of the norm.[2]

In my opinion, EMDR can help victims of childhood sexual and physical abuse to reclaim the sense of self that was once violated and long silenced. Additional information about EMDR is provided in the resources section at the conclusion of this case report.

- Consultation with the counselor at her school, who would honor GG's request for confidentiality.

- Participation in a martial arts training program offered at her school, which would help GG to create mental and physical self-survival strategies.

☞ **Cinematherapy**
- *Monsoon Wedding*

- *Wall Street* (1987)

- *Whale Rider*

☞ Suggested reading to share with a trustworthy teacher or school counselor

Bolen JS. *Ring of Power: The Abandoned Child, the Authoritarian Father, and the Disempowered Feminine : A Jungian Understanding of Wagner's Ring Cycle*. San Francisco, Calif: HarperSanFrancisco; 1992.

Sanford LT. *Strong At the Broken Places: Overcoming the Trauma of Childhood Abuse*. New York, NY: Random House; 1990.

☞ Internet resource

www.emdr.org — EMDR Institute, Inc - Information on eye movement desensitization and reprocessing (EMDR)

Follow Up

Eventually, GG developed a trusting relationship with a counselor and began the path to recovery.

Discussion

The sexual trauma or physical abuse of girls profoundly and negatively affects their future emotional health status. Health status and lifestyle choices are adversely affected by childhood trauma. Women and adolescent survivors of childhood abuse are more likely to experience depression, anxiety, eating disorders, insomnia, obesity, self-destructive or suicidal impulses, chronic headaches, substance abuse, sexual dysfunction, gastrointestinal complaints, fibromyalgia, pelvic pain, somatization disorder, fluctuating high blood pressure, and asthma.[3,4] Although the medical literature supports those associations, physicians are unlikely to inquire about such trauma during the physician-patient interaction.

Adult survivors of childhood trauma are often unrecognized by their physicians because no clearcut characteristics serve as red flags for that type of abuse. Research has revealed that most patients appreciate being asked about experiences of prior victimization because they believe that their physician can help with associated emotional or physical problems.[5,6]

We as physicians must be aware of the alarming incidence of childhood abuse, and we must be certain to include sensitive, emotionally supportive, and appropriate inquiries about such experiences as part of patient care. As in the case of GG, an urgent appointment for headache treatment may really be a call for a different kind of help.

References

1. Rothbaum BO. A controlled study of eye movement desensitization and reprocessing in the treatment of posttraumatic stress disordered sexual assault victims. *Bull Menninger Clin.* 1997;61(3):317-334.

2. Scheck MM, Schaeffer JA, Gillette C. Brief psychological intervention with traumatized young women: the efficacy of eye movement desensitization and reprocessing. *J Trauma Stress.* 1998;11(1):25-44.

3. Bolen JD. The impact of sexual abuse on women's health. *Psych Annals.* 1993;23(8):446-453.

4. Laws A. Sexual abuse history and women's medical problems. *J Gen Intern Med.* 1993;8(8):441-443.

5. Friedman LS, Samet JH, Roberts MS, Hudlin M, Hans P. Inquiry about victimization experiences. A survey of patient preferences and physician practices. *Arch Intern Med.* 1992;152(6):1186-1190.

6. Butterfield MI, Bastian LA, McIntyre LM, et al. Screening for mental disorders and history of sexual trauma and battering among women using primary health care services. *JCOM.* 1996;3(5):55-60.

Case 8. Giving Up

HH, a 16-year-old female patient, had been in my care for several years. I had only treated her for minor illnesses and performed her physical examinations for school. However, I received a call from a nurse in the psychiatric unit of our facility, who informed me that HH had been admitted to the hospital because she had taken an overdose of Tylenol. I was aware of recent stresses in HH's family because her mother was also my patient. When I visited HH in her hospital room, she stated that she had taken the overdose because she "wanted to die, to get out and get away." She also said, however, that she had told her sister shortly after she had taken the overdose, and her sister had called for help.

HH was the older of 2 daughters. When she was hospitalized, she was living with her biologic parents and younger sister and attended a public high school. She was intelligent and good-natured, and she had bright blue eyes and a petite build. She said that in the past few months, her world had changed dramatically. Her parents were divorcing because they were deeply in debt and her mother's addiction to cocaine had become unbearable. HH's father had decided to file for custody of the children. She said that her car had been sold and she had had to stop her extracurricular activities to get a job at a fast-food restaurant to help defray family expenses. Those changes in her life prevented her from being with friends. Her excellent grades had begun to decline because she could not concentrate when she was depressed.

At the time of her hospitalization, HH was being treated with no medications, she had undergone no prior surgeries, and she had suffered no major illnesses. Her menstrual periods, which had begun when she was 13 years of age, occurred every 28 to 32 days. Although HH had been sexually active, she was not involved in a sexual relationship at that time. Her father and siblings were healthy, but her maternal grandfather had abused alcohol. HH had recently started smoking cigarettes to get breaks at work. She denied alcohol or drug use and had lost 5 pounds since her last office visit 3 months previously.

Diagnosis
Depression with suicide attempt

☞ Treatment

I referred HH to a psychotherapist and to Al-Anon, an organization for friends and family members of individuals addicted to alcohol or drugs. I also advised her to seek support from her extended family. We discussed whether she could decrease her work hours, which would enable her to participate in at least 1 school activity. I suggested that she select a favorite teacher as her mentor or advisor so that she could discuss her feelings honestly and without inhibition and could be guided in setting new academic and social goals. I also recommended that HH:

- Continue to receive psychiatric care and psychotherapy as initiated in the psychiatric unit of the hospital in which she had been treated.

- Practice yoga to assist in stress management and improve her mood (see Chapter 3).

- Schedule a Bio-Touch session for stress management at least once weekly (more often if needed). I also suggested that HH could teach the Bio-Touch technique to her younger sister so that they could help each other (See Chapter 7).

- Complete a handwork project (see Chapter 5).

☞ Cinematherapy
- *Boost*

- *What's Eating Gilbert Grape?*

- *The Breakfast Club*

Follow Up

At the time of her 4-week follow-up visit, HH had made some changes in her life. She said that attending Al-Anon meetings had been very helpful because she had met other teens who were experiencing challenges similar to her own. She reported that her mood was more stable, and she was optimistic about her future.

Discussion

In the United States, depression in adolescents is twice as prevalent in girls as in boys.[1] Almost all teens periodically exhibit mood swings, melancholy, or low mood, but clinical depression is a different problem. It is a much more serious despair that is characterized by the following symptoms, which persist for more than 2 weeks: sad or irritable mood; a loss of interest or pleasure in formerly enjoyable activities; a change in appetite, weight, activity, energy level, or sleep habits; expressions of self-reproach or inappropriate guilt; difficulty in concentrating; and suicidal thoughts or gestures like that made by HH.[1]

Evidence has shown that psychotherapy is helpful in the treatment of adolescent depression. However, recent controversy about antidepressant use in children and teenagers has been featured in the headlines of lay publications and in the medical literature.[2] In fact, the United Kingdom recently banned the use of such medications in children and adolescents.[3]

Emotional resilience (the ability to effectively manage adversity, trauma, tragedy, and similar stressors) can be taught by a caring adult, a parent, another family member, a friend, or a teacher. People who learn to be resilient can set achievable goals; nurture their self-esteem; adhere to a daily structure and routine; accept the necessity of change; relate to others through friendships, volunteer activities, or community group functions; overcome difficult situations at home, at work, or at school; talk about their mistakes; openly express disappointment; and accept change as part of growing up.

Adolescent women are especially vulnerable to mood disorders and suicide because they are subject to extreme hormonal changes and associated neurologic and physical effects that can be exacerbated by emotional stress. Valuing peer relationships over family interactions renders some teens less willing to talk with their parents about fears and uncertainties.

Bethany Hamilton, the 13-year-old surfer who survived a horrific shark attack but lost an arm, is a tribute to youthful resilience and an inspiration to girls and young women.[4] She reacted to her loss with altruism, humor, and optimism, and even asked that the life of the shark that attacked her be spared.

References

1. Tancer NK, Shaffer D. Depression. In: Friedman SB, Fisher M, Schonberg SK, eds. *Comprehensive Adolescent Health Care*. St. Louis, Mo: Quality Medical Publishing Inc; 1992.

2. Breggin PR. Suicidality, violence and mania caused by selective serotonin reuptake inhibitors (SSRIs): a review and analysis. *Intnl J Risk Safety Med*. 2003/2004;16:31-49.

3. Healy D, Whitaker C. Antidepressants and suicide: risk-benefit conundrums. *J Psychiatry Neurosci*. 2003;28(5):331-337.

4. Lieber J. Hamilton an inspiration to others after losing arm. *USA Today*. March 19, 2004:C15.

Case 9. System Overload

VV, a 16-year-old patient who lived with her parents, sought treatment for multiple symptoms. She complained of irregular menstrual periods that occurred every 26 to 45 days. She also experienced fatigue and had difficulty awakening in the morning and falling asleep at night. According to her mother, VV experienced mood swings more frequently than she had in the past, and she had difficulty concentrating. VV said that she craved sugar and had noticed a recent weight gain around her waist.

She did not smoke. Although she occasionally consumed alcohol, she denied other drug use.

VV attended a public high school and was a member of the high school honor society. She drove her own car. She mentioned that academic pressure, the demands of a part-time job at a fast-food restaurant, and family conflicts had increased her level of emotional stress. She reported skipping breakfast, eating lunch at the school cafeteria, and eating evening meals at the fast food restaurant or at home.

At the time of her examination, VV was treating her headaches as needed with a combination analgesic (Excedrin) containing aspirin, acetaminophen, and caffeine. She reported no prior illnesses or surgeries and was not sexually active. Her menstrual periods had begun when she was 11 years of age. Her mother and father were overweight, and her siblings, whose weight was within a normal range, were healthy. Her maternal grandmother was diabetic and had high blood pressure. One aunt suffered from polycystic ovary syndrome and diabetes, and one cousin was diagnosed as having polycystic ovary syndrome.

VV's physical examination revealed acne on her face, chest, back, and upper arms and excess hair on her face, thighs, and lower abdomen. She was overweight. Her blood pressure was elevated. Serum and saliva testing revealed the following results:

Serum testing (range)
 Thyroid hormones: Normal
 High-density lipoprotein cholesterol (HDL): Low
 Triglycerides: High
 Insulin: High
 Glucose: Above normal

Saliva testing (range)
>Estradiol: Normal
>Progesterone: Low
>Progesterone-estradiol ratio: Low
>Testosterone: High
>Dehydroepiandrosterone sulfate (DHEAS): High
>Cortisol: Morning - Normal
>>Bedtime - High

Pelvic ultrasonography revealed small cysts on both ovaries.

Diagnosis

Polycystic ovary syndrome (PCOS), metabolic syndrome, adrenal dysfunction

☞ Treatment

To treat VV's hormone imbalances, I prescribed the following therapy:

- Bioidentical progesterone cream 40 mg/mL (0.5 mL to be applied at bedtime to a thin-skinned area such as the inner arm or inner thigh for the first 10 days of the menstrual cycle; then 1 mL to be applied to a different thin-skinned area at bedtime from day 11 until the start of menstruation) (see Chapter 6).

- A topical antibiotic for the treatment of acne.

- A multivitamin with B complex and vitamins C and E.

- Chromium picolinate 400 mcg 3 times daily.

- Following the Mediterranean diet, which is practical for the teenage lifestyle; foods can be eaten "on the go" or carried in a back pack.

- Avoiding sugar and high-carbohydrate, high-fat foods.

- Participating in an exercise program offered by her high school.

- Practicing yoga to help to balance hormone levels (see Chapter 3).

- A Bio-Touch session once weekly to reduce stress (see Chapter 7).

- Completing a handwork project (see Chapter 5).

 Cinematherapy
- *Breaking Away*

- *October Sky*

 Suggested reading
Wilson JL. *Adrenal Fatigue: The 21st Century Stress Syndrome.* Petaluma, Calif: Smart Publications; 2001. — A source of excellent information on low-glycemic diets. Web site: www.adrenalfatigue.org.

 Internet resource
www.oldwayspt.org — Information about the Mediterranean diet.

Follow Up

At VV's 8-week follow-up visit, the results of laboratory testing revealed that her levels of insulin, progesterone, glucose, KDL, triglycerides, and testosterone were in the normal range and that her morning level of cortisol had improved. VV reported 2 normal menstrual cycles. She noted fewer headaches, mood swings, and food cravings and was less fatigued. Her quality of sleep had improved, as had her acne. She had lost 7 pounds. She was exercising sporadically but had made significant dietary changes.

Discussion

PCOS can develop at any time during a woman's reproductive life and even during menopause. It is a syndrome characterized by irregular menstrual periods; midbody weight gain; increased facial hair; elevated blood pressure; acne; infertility; an excess of androgens, testosterone, and dehydroepiandrosterone (DHEA); and an underproduction of progesterone. It is strongly associated with metabolic syndrome, which is characterized by insulin resistance that increases as a result of a sedentary lifestyle, smoking, a high level of stress, excessive consumption of carbohydrates, obesity, and/or treatment with synthetic hormone replacement. In my clinical experience, PCOS is occurring more often in young women than it did 15 years ago, probably as a result of several factors: our stressful modern lifestyle; increased fast-food consumption; a diet high in sugar, fats, and carbohydrates; and inactivity. Untreated PCOS can increase the risk of diabetes and cardiovascular disease.[1]

Reference

1. Wise DE, Dewester J. Metabolic syndrome and associated cardiovascular disease risk. *Am Acad Fam Physicians. CME Bulletin.* 2004;3(2):1-5.

Case 10. Overstressed and Overeating

JJ, a 21-year-old woman with multiple physical and emotional symptoms, sought my help. She suffered from mood swings that ranged from anxious and depressed to aggressive and angry. She also reported unexplained fatigue; a craving for sweets, bread, and salt; joint pain; bloating; thinning scalp hair; acne; intolerance to cold; and tension-related headaches. Her cognitive symptoms included uncharacteristic forgetfulness, difficulty in concentrating, and difficulty in decision making. She often responded to emotional stress by binge eating, after which she used laxatives, exercise, or fasting to avoid weight gain.

JJ had begun to menstruate at 12 years of age, and her menstrual periods occurred every 28 to 32 days until she was 16 or 17 years old. At that time, her menstrual cycle became irregular, and she sometimes did not menstruate for 2 or 3 months between cycles. She was not sexually active.

During high school, JJ had experienced clinical depression for which she was hospitalized and treated with medication. Her medical history was otherwise unremarkable, and she had undergone no surgeries. She reported taking over-the-counter preparations (acetaminophen [Tylenol] or naproxen sodium [Aleve]) to treat her headaches. Her parents were overweight, and her mother suffered from hypothyroidism. Her siblings were healthy.

JJ lived with both biologic parents and her siblings. She was a full-time college student and worked part-time on campus. Her academic performance was superior. She denied the use of alcohol, tobacco, or illicit drugs. She exercised to compensate for overeating and followed a low-fat, low-calorie diet except when she was binge eating.

Physical examination revealed a thin young woman with blood pressure in the normal range; dry, thinning scalp hair; acne of the face, chest, and back; increased hair distribution on the face, arms, thighs, and lower abdomen; and hands and feet that were cool to the touch. Serum and saliva testing revealed the following results:

Serum testing (range)
Thyroid-stimulating hormone (TSH): High normal
Levothyroxine (T_4): Low normal
Basic metabolic panel (blood chemistry panel): Normal
Complete blood count: Normal

Saliva testing (range)
>   Estradiol: Slightly low
>   Progesterone: Low
>   Progesterone-estradiol ratio: Low
>   Testosterone: High
>   Dehydroepiandrosterone sulfate (DHEAS): High
>   Cortisol: Morning - High
>>   Noon - Low
>>   Evening - High
>>   Bedtime - Low

Diagnosis

Androgen excess, progesterone deficiency, adrenal dysfunction, bulimia, characteristics of rapid aging, functional hypothyroidism, obsessive-compulsive personality traits manifested as perfectionism

☞ *Treatment*

To correct JJ's hormone imbalances, I prescribed the following treatment:

- Bioidentical progesterone cream 40 mg/mL (0.5 mL to be applied once daily to a thin-skinned area, such as the inner arm or inner thigh, at bedtime for 10 days; then the same amount twice daily [in the morning and again at bedtime] to a different thin-skinned area until the start of menstruation). Progesterone decreases the level of testosterone, DHEAS, and cortisol at the tissue level (see Chapter 6).

- Armour thyroid tablets, USP, for once-daily oral administration in the morning (15 mg for 3 weeks; then 30 mg daily).

- A multivitamin with B complex and vitamins E and C once daily.

- An antibiotic to treat acne vulgaris.

- Adhering to the Mediterranean diet.

- Practicing yoga 3 to 5 times weekly (see Chapter 3).

- Completing a handwork project (see Chapter 5).

- Scheduling a Bio-Touch session once weekly to reduce stress (see Chapter 7).

- Volunteering for a nonacademic worthy cause to foster social interaction.

☞ Cinematherapy
- *Broadcast News*

- *Good Will Hunting*

☞ Suggested reading
Wilson JL. *Adrenal Fatigue: The 21st Century Stress Syndrome*. Petaluma, Calif: Smart Publications; 2001. Web site: www.adrenalfatigue.org.

Borysenko J. *Guilt Is the Teacher, Love Is the Lesson*. New York, NY: Warner Books; 1990.

☞ Internet resources
www.mirasol.net/index.html — Mirasol is a facility in Tucson, Arizona, that offers a treatment program for eating disorders.

www.nationaleatingdisorders.org — The National Eating Disorders Association.

www.oldwayspt.org — Information about the Mediterranean diet.

Follow Up
At her 8-week follow-up examination, JJ reported attending yoga class or practicing yoga 4 to 5 times per week. She said that she had a greater awareness of the effects of emotional stress in her life and that she had improved her ability to cope with those issues. She had noted a

new growth of scalp hair and said that her hair texture had improved and her skin seemed less dry. Her fatigue had resolved, and her joint pain was markedly diminished. She reported experiencing fewer food cravings, headaches, and mood swings. Her acne was also resolving. Her TSH and T_4 levels were within normal ranges. Saliva testing revealed that JJ's estradiol level was in the low-normal range; her progesterone, testosterone, and DHEAS levels were near normal values; and the daily rhythm of her cortisol levels had improved.

Discussion

Ninety percent of the estimated 8 million people in the United States who have an eating disorder are women.[1] Eating disorders, which occur in all ethnic and socioeconomic groups, usually begin during adolescence but have been reported in children as young as 8 years.

Bulimia is an eating disorder characterized by the consumption of a large amount of food in a short period of time (binging), which is followed by laxative use, vomiting, fasting, or extreme exercising to prevent weight gain. Bulimic individuals, who may be of normal weight, too thin, or obese, have a preoccupation with food and with their weight. They often conceal their eating patterns. A low level of estrogen, an elevated testosterone level, and normal or lean body weight have been associated with bulimia.[2]

I have noted that bulimic individuals sometimes experience rapid aging, which also is associated with a high stress level, poor diet, a high or low level of testosterone, and abnormal cortisol levels that vary during a 24-hour period. In those suffering from bulimia, the results of serum thyroid hormone evaluations may be within the normal range or borderline, but the symptoms of thyroid hormone deficiency are nonetheless evident and patients respond favorably to thyroid supplementation.

References

1. National Association of Anorexia Nervosa and Associated Disorders Web site. Available at: www.nationaleatingdisorders.org. Accessed July 1, 2004.

2. Rohr UD. The impact of testosterone imbalance on depression and women's health. *Maturitas.* 2002;41(suppl 1):S25-S46.

Case 11. Progesterone, Not Prozac

KK, a 25-year-old female patient, complained of worsening premenstrual syndrome (PMS). She described multiple symptoms (depressed mood, irritability, a feeling of being overwhelmed and very stressed, a craving for sugar, bloating, breast tenderness, decreased stamina, aches and pains, fatigue [especially during the morning], difficulty in falling asleep and in concentrating) that she noted during the second half of her menstrual cycle. Those symptoms significantly affected her work, social activities, and relationships. Treatment with St. John's wort and several over-the-counter medications for PMS had been ineffective, and she was not being treated with other medications.

KK had begun to menstruate at the age of 12 years. Her menstrual periods, which occurred regularly every 28 to 32 days, lasted for about 5 days. She was sexually active infrequently and used condoms for contraception. Her mother had been diagnosed as having hypothyroidism, her father was alive and well, and her siblings were healthy.

KK had a college degree and was employed full-time. She lived alone in an apartment. She had not exercised for 1 year because the demands of her job had increased and she had little leisure time. Her diet consisted of pastries for breakfast, fast food for lunch, and microwavable entrees for dinner. She consumed 4 to 6 caffeinated beverages per day except during episodes of PMS, when she increased her caffeine consumption to relieve fatigue. She drank 3 to 5 alcoholic beverages per week during episodes of PMS and did not smoke or use illicit drugs. She had a circle of supportive friends and saw her parents at least once each month.

KK's medical history was unremarkable. She had undergone no surgical procedures and had no current illnesses, but she was clinically overweight. Serum and saliva testing revealed the following results:

Serum testing (range)
  Thyroid hormones: Normal

Saliva testing (range)
  Estradiol: Normal
  Progesterone: Low
  Progesterone - estradiol ratio: Low
  Testosterone: Normal
  Dehydroepiandrosterone sulfate (DHEAS): Normal
  Cortisol: Morning - Low normal
          Bedtime - Low normal

Diagnosis
Progesterone deficiency, premenstrual dysphoric disorder (PMDD)

☞ Treatment
I suggested the following regimen as treatment for KK's hormone imbalance:

  - Bioidentical progesterone extended-release tablets (see the discussion on hormones and the formulary in Chapter 6) 300 mg (one-half tablet at bedtime on the first day of menstruation through cycle day 10, then 1 tablet 2 to 4 times daily on day 11 of the menstrual cycle, a dosage to be continued until the start of menstruation).

- A calcium supplement with magnesium and a multivitamin containing vitamin B complex.

- A gradual decrease in caffeine intake to 2 beverages daily.

- A reduction in alcohol and salt intake.

- An increase in protein consumption (goal: one-third of daily calories from protein).

- Preparing meals at home at least 3 evenings per week.

- Participation in an aerobic-exercise program (brisk walking, running, cycling, dancing, swimming) 3 to 5 days weekly for 20 to 30 minutes.

- Practicing yoga 1 to 3 times weekly (see Chapter 3).

- Completing a handwork project (see Chapter 5).

- Scheduling a Biotouch session once weekly for stress reduction (see Chapter 7).

- Taking a cooking class, which is a wonderful way to improve diet and to learn about meal preparation.

Follow Up
At the time of her 8-week follow-up visit, KK reported a marked improvement in all symptoms. She had lost 7 pounds and had experienced no adverse effects from treatment with progesterone. She felt best when she took 3 tablets of the prescribed dosage of progesterone per day

(morning, afternoon, and bedtime) during the second half of her menstrual cycle. She had joined a health club near her workplace and was exercising 5 days per week. Follow-up saliva testing revealed that all hormone levels were within the normal range as a result of progesterone supplementation.

Discussion

My husband and I are Monday-night football fans. At a commercial break during a game a few years ago, I was infuriated when I saw a television commercial announcing the availability of Sarafem, which is a form of fluoxetine (Prozac). The ad portrayed a young woman who was overly emotional, out of control, and incapacitated. Her husband looked helpless as she went on a premenstrual rampage through the house. After treatment with Sarafem, the same woman was portrayed as charming, attractive, and being emotionally engaged with her husband and children. Shortly after the release of that commercial, requests for Sarafem from my patients and/or their husbands soared. The long arm of the pharmaceutical companies was again successful in reaching a receptive audience and pathologizing women who, it was suggested, could be instantly cured by treatment with a psychiatric drug.

PMS, which refers to the physical discomfort and/or mood changes that occur during the menstrual cycle, affects 40% to 70% of women who menstrate.[1] However, most women are not incapacitated by PMS; they effectively compensate and plan for the anticipated fluctuation of their hormone levels. Research has shown that premenstrual symptoms do not include measurable cognitive dysfunction or a decrease in intellectual performance, reaction time, or attention span.[2]

Only about 3% to 8 % of American women experience PMDD (a more severe form of PMS), despite advertisements suggesting that the disorder is common.[3] Unfortunately, irritable women are often quickly labeled as suffering from PMDD, and many physicians hold the prescription pen ready. The science of selling trumps the scientific evidence.

The diagnosis of PMDD is based on 3 factors:

1. The symptoms appear in the second half of the menstrual cycle and resolve when menstruation begins or a few days thereafter.

2. The symptoms are severe enough to markedly interfere with work, social activities, and/or relationships.

3. No psychiatric or physical cause for the symptoms is identified.

Some physicians prescribe potent antipsychotic drugs to treat PMS or PMDD. In my medical training, I was directed to liberally prescribe antianxiety drugs such as alprazolam (Xanax), lorazepam (Ativan), or diazepam (Valium) or antidepressants such as fluoxetine (Prozac) for the treatment of those disorders. As I began to study and investigate further, however, I concluded that PMDD and PMS are caused by too little progesterone in the second half of the menstrual cycle.[4]

To minimize the symptoms of PMS, I recommend nutritional changes such as consuming a maximum of 2 caffeine-containing beverages per day and avoiding alcohol and salt. I also suggest taking calcium and magnesium supplements and increasing the level of exercise. Stress reduction and schedule changes can be tailored to the patient's symptoms. For example, if the need for sleep is greater during the second half of the menstrual cycle, I encourage the patient to plan weekend naps or to start her work day later during that time, if possible.

I have found that bioidentical progesterone supplementation is very effective in relieving the symptoms of PMDD and PMS in patients who have a hormone imbalance. Progesterone is a neuroactive hormone; it exerts a powerful effect on the neurotransmitters in the brain used to convey naturally psychotropic substances that relieve anxiety and depression, food cravings, and irritability, which are common symptoms of PMDD and PMS. Progesterone also alleviates bloating, fluid retention, sleep disturbance, and breast tenderness (see Chapter 6 on hormones).[5]

I usually prescribe oral bioidentical progesterone initially to relieve PMDD or PMS because it exerts a calming, sedating, and stabilizing effect on mood. If patients find oral progesterone too sedating, I prescribe that hormone as a cream. Some patients find that a combination of oral and topical progesterone is most effective.

By treating the hormone imbalance rather than symptoms, it is possible to avoid the adverse effects of potent antianxiety drugs, antidepressants, and antipsychotic medications and to prevent the detrimental labeling of the patient as having a primary psychiatric disorder. One of my patients was recently denied life insurance because she was taking an antidepressant drug for a nonpsychiatric condition. Even though she presented documentation that confirmed her physical disorder, her insurance application was denied. Her husband, who was a smoker, was able to obtain a life insurance policy without difficulty.

References

1. Johnson SR, McChesney C, Bean JA. Epidemiology of premenstrual symptoms in a nonclinical sample. I. Prevalence, natural history and help-seeking behavior. *J Reprod Med.* 1988;33(4):340-346.

2. Morgan M, Rapkin A. Cognitive flexibility, reaction time, and attention in women with premenstrual dysphoric disorder. *J Gend Specif Med.* 2002;5(3):28-36.

3. Rivera-Tovar AD, Frank E. Late luteal phase dysphoric disorder in young women. *Am J Psychiatry.* 1990;147(12):1634-1636.

4. Dalton K. *The Premenstrual Syndrome and Progesterone Therapy.* 2nd ed. London, England: William Heinemann Medical Books; 1984.

5. Rupprecht R, Holsboer F. Neuroactive steroids: mechanisms of action and neuropsychopharmacological perspectives. *Trends Neurosci.* 1999;22(9):410-416.

Case 12. Too Tired to Cook

LL, a 26-year-old patient, requested evaluation after noting a report of increased blood pressure obtained from a blood pressure machine at a drug store. Her symptoms, which had worsened over the past 2 years, included palpitations, dizziness, weight gain, acne, a craving for sugar, mood swings, migraines, and irregular menstrual periods.

At the time of her appointment, LL was being treated with sumatriptan (Imitrex) to relieve migraine and loratadine (Claritin) to alleviate allergic rhinitis. She had undergone tubal ligation and had experienced 3 pregnancies, 2 of which had culminated in normal deliveries and 1 in miscarriage. Her mother suffered from depression, her father's health status was unknown, and her siblings were healthy. Her maternal grandmother had died of a heart attack, and her maternal grandfather had high blood pressure.

LL was a single mother of 2 children who were 4 and 6 years of age. Both children were overweight. LL was employed full-time at a desk job that required using a computer all day. She did not exercise. She denied tobacco and alcohol use but stated that she drank two to three 64-oz sugar-containing sodas daily. She said that she was "too tired to cook" and that her children "only eat fast food anyway." She reported a high stress level caused by conflicts with her ex-husband, pressure from work, and financial problems.

LL suffered from abdominal obesity and facial acne. Physical examination revealed that her blood pressure was slightly elevated. Serum and saliva testing revealed the following results:

Serum testing (range)
      Insulin: Normal
      Glucose: Normal
      Triglycerides: Normal
      Cholesterol: Normal
      Thyroid hormones: Normal

Saliva testing (range):
      Estradiol: Normal
      Progesterone: Low
      Progesterone-estradiol ratio: Low
      Testosterone: High
      Dehydroepiandrosterone sulfate (DHEAS): High

Diagnosis

Estrogen dominance, progesterone deficiency, androgen excess, obesity, mild high blood pressure

☞ **Treatment**
- Bioidentical progesterone 300 mg (1 tablet at bedtime on days 1 to 10 of the menstrual cycle, then 1 tablet 2 to 4 times daily on cycle days 11 to 28) (see Chapter 6).

- Oral and topical antibiotics for the treatment of facial acne.

- Replacing the consumption of sugar-containing soda with diet soda, which would then be gradually eliminated from LL's diet.

- Decreasing fast-food consumption to 3 times weekly.

- Beginning an exercise program on her lunch-hour break at work.

- Practicing yoga at home with her children 1 to 3 times weekly (see Chapter 3).

- Participating with her children in the Kid's Workshop, a program offered nationwide by Home Depot. Children 12 years of age or younger join a parent or guardian (2 children per adult) on the first Saturday of each month to build and complete a project (a soapbox derby car, a bird house, a kaleidoscope, etc). There is no charge for the workshop, and all materials (including an apron for each child) are free. Contact a local Home Depot for more information about the Kid's Workshop (see Chapter 5).

- Scheduling a Bio-Touch session once weekly (see Chapter 7).

- Joining a TOPS (Take Off Pounds Sensibly) support group.

☞ *Cinematherapy*
- *One Fine Day* (1996)

☞ Suggested reading

Spangel L. *Life Is Hard, Food Is Easy: The 5-Step Plan to Overcome Emotional Eating and Lose Weight on Any Diet.* Washington, DC; Lanham, Md: Lifeline Press; 2003.

Schlosser E. *Fast Food Nation: The Dark Side of the All-American Meal.* Boston, Mass: Houghton Mifflin; 2001.

Kabat-Zinn M, Kabat-Zinn J. *Everyday Blessings: The Inner Work of Mindful Parenting.* New York, NY: Hyperion; 1997.

☞ Internet resource

www.tops.org — TOPS (Take Off Pounds Sensibly) support group.

Follow Up

At her 8-week follow-up appointment, LL reported no adverse effects from treatment with bioidentical progesterone. She had more energy and had begun 2 types of exercise: a walking program on the stairs and in the parking lot at work and yoga practice via video instruction at home. LL said that she was enjoying the experience of preparing some meals at home with her children. She had become more aware of emotional patterns that increased her desire to eat and was experiencing a more even overall mood. Her facial acne was resolving, and she had lost 10 pounds.

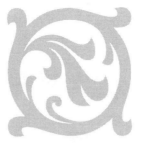

Appendix B:
Case Reports — Adulthood
to Midlife

Athena, the Greek goddess of war and wisdom, was considered the inventor of many practical items such as the chariot, the flute, the earthenware pot, the plough, the rake, and the ship. She was the teacher of the science of numbers and all women's arts, such as cooking, weaving, and spinning. A fierce warrior, she could also change her appearance to assist or protect others or to defend herself against attack. Women from 30 to 60 years of age (the group featured in this chapter) experience heightened physical and emotional demands. They often exhibit the Athenian traits of being able to invent, adapt, create, and change in response to the needs of family or friends. Many women in the second phase of the feminine life cycle demonstrate great passion for a cause or career. They also know the importance of honoring their own need for regeneration and respite from emotional turmoil and feel the tension between their outer persona, which they present to the world, and their inner self, which may remain veiled. In response to that tension, many women in midlife shed the burden of guilt, fear, or obligation and transform into their authentic self, which may mean leaving a career, a marriage, or a relationship and embarking on the quest to realize their lost dreams.

This chapter is dedicated to Mara B, who has demonstrated the Athenian ideal of emotional resilience after facing the challenges of raising a special-needs child, serving as a caregiver to a parent with Alzheimer's disease, experiencing the death of a parent, and facing the greatest of all losses — the death of a child. Despite those traumas, Mara, like Athena, has been trustworthy and responsible. She has sustained and nurtured a long-lasting marriage, continued volunteer work for socioeconomically disadvantaged families, maintained an antiques business, served as surrogate matriarch in her extended family, and been a loyal and loving sister, cousin, aunt, and daughter-in-law and a supportive, loving friend who is sought for her wise counsel and knowledge.

The following case reports describe the health challenges of and therapies for women in the middle third of life — those who live the Athenian ideals of truth to oneself and devotion to others.

Case 1. Too Old Too Soon

AA, a 35-year-old woman, sought consultation about a constellation of symptoms that she had experienced during the prior 12 months of declining health. Her symptoms included thin, dry hair; persistent, unrelieved fatigue; dry skin; brown patches on her face; a weight gain of 30 pounds over 12 months; leg cramps; premenstrual headaches; aches and pains; severe bloating; difficulty with word and name retrieval; short-term memory loss; decreased libido; and mood swings. She had been evaluated by her primary care physician, an internist, 2 obstetrician-gynecologists, an endocrinologist, and a psychiatrist. Oral contraceptives, antidepressants, and antianxiety medications had been ineffective in relieving her symptoms. She denied alcohol or tobacco use.

At the time of her examination in our clinic, AA was being treated with albuterol sulfate (Proventil) via inhaler as needed for occasional mild asthma attacks and ibuprofen as needed to treat aches and pains. Her menstrual periods occurred every 28 to 30 days. She had experienced 2 normal pregnancies with nominal deliveries of healthy infants. Her last child was born 18 months before her visit to our clinic. AA had undergone no prior surgeries. Her mother, father, and siblings were healthy. High blood pressure, diabetes, and heart disease afflicted her extended family members.

AA was married and lived with her spouse and 2 children. She worked full-time in health care. She had managed to fulfill her job responsibilities during the preceding months but stated that she "collapsed" after returning home from work, when she immediately went to bed until she arose for work the next morning. She felt guilty about not being available for her children's needs and placing the burden of housework, meals, laundry, and other houschold chores on her husband.

Physical examination revealed that AA was obese. Her complexion was dull; her skin, thin; and her scalp hair, thin and greying. Bone density testing revealed osteopenia (decreased bone density). Her responses to standard tests of depression and anxiety were within the normal range. Serum and saliva testing revealed the following results:

Serum testing (range)
   Thyroid hormones: Normal

Saliva testing (range)
> Estradiol: Low
> Progesterone: Low
> Progesterone-estradiol ratio: Low
> Testosterone: Low
> Dehydroepiandrosterone sulfate (DHEAS): Low
> Cortisol: Morning - Low
> > Noon - Low
> > Evening - Low
> > Bedtime - Low

Diagnosis

Deficiencies of estrogen, progesterone, testosterone, and dehydroepiandrosterone (DHEA); adrenal exhaustion; functional hypothyroidism; rapid aging

☞ Treatment

- A capsule containing a combination of the following bioidentical hormones: 80% estriol and 20% estradiol (Bi-Est, 1.25 mg) plus testosterone 4 mg in oil (1 capsule by mouth each morning) (see Chapter 6).

- Bioidentical progesterone 300 mg (1 extended-release tablet at bedtime on days 1 to 9 of the menstrual cycle, then 1 tablet 2 to 4 times daily on cycle days 10 to 28) (see Chapter 6).

- Thyroid tablets, USP (Armour thyroid) 15 mg (1 tablet daily).

- Adherence to the Mediterranean diet (see Internet resources below).

- A calcium supplement containing vitamin D and a multivitamin containing vitamins C and E once daily.

- Practicing "bedtop" yoga 4 to 5 times weekly (see Chapter 3).

- Keeping a diary of symptoms.

- Scheduling a Bio-Touch session once weekly (see Chapter 7).

- Completing a handwork project (see Chapter 5). For patients like AA, whose household productivity has been diminished because of profound physical and emotional changes, the ability to begin and complete a simple handwork project can bring a much-needed sense of accomplishment and induce relaxation.

☞ **Suggested reading**
Vliet EL. *Screaming To Be Heard! Hormonal Connections Women Suspect — and Doctors Ignore.* New York, NY: M. Evans and Co; 1995.

Wilson JL. *Adrenal Fatigue: The 21st Century Stress Syndrome.* Petaluma, Calif: Smart Publications; 2001. Web site: www.adrenalfatigue.org.

☞ **Recommended resources for bedtop yoga practice**
Dickman C. Bed Top Yoga [video]. Studio name not available; 1999.

Dickman C. Bed Top Yoga. 1st edition [audio cassette]. Yoga Enterprises; 1997.

☞ **Internet resources**
www.oldwayspt.org — Information about the Mediterranean diet.

www.stretch.com — Information about bedtop yoga.

Follow Up

At her 8-week follow-up appointment, AA reported an overall improvement in her health. She felt rested when she awoke and had the energy to accomplish several household tasks after her work day. She had experienced fewer headaches, aches, and pains and noted less bloating, more moisture in her hair and skin, and increased stamina. She felt best when she took progesterone in the prescribed dosage 4 times daily during the second half of her menstrual cycle.

Secondary Follow Up

At her 16-week follow-up, AA reported having regular monthly menstrual periods. She was engaging in aerobic exercise for 30 minutes 6 days per week and had enrolled in a yoga class. She had experienced no headaches and noted fewer food cravings. She had lost 25 pounds and had noted an improvement in the texture of her hair and skin. Her libido had improved. Her level of intellectual functioning had returned to normal, and she reported having no problem with concentration or memory. The results of saliva testing for hormone imbalance were within the normal range. AA stated that she felt well enough to host a social event in her home during the following month.

Discussion

I have treated a number of women like AA who have sought help from several physicians for an unexplained constellation of symptoms. Hormonal imbalances can occur even in patients whose menstrual cycle is normal. Rapid aging is diagnosed when a patient exhibits physical signs and symptoms that are more often observed in older individuals. I have observed that rapid aging is strongly associated with hormonal imbalance (including an abnormal cortisol pattern) and is intensified by a high stress level, a sedentary lifestyle, and a diet high in fat and sugar. Treatment with bioidentical hormone replacement therapy (BHRT) and healthful changes in lifestyle enable such patients to return to their previous level of greater activity and good health.

Case 2. Grief from Loss

BB, a patient in her late 30s, requested an appointment for the evaluation of headache pain. However, during her examination she stated that she had not been experiencing headaches but that several times daily she was experiencing rapid heartbeat, shortness of breath, chest tightness, and difficulty in concentrating and sleeping. Those symptoms had been present for several weeks. I asked BB if she had experienced any changes or stressors several weeks ago, and she hesitated. She then stated that her husband had a fertility problem and that they had saved enough money to pay for in vitro fertilization. In that procedure, eggs taken from BB's ovaries were to be fertilized with her husband's sperm in the laboratory to form an embryo. The resultant embryos (usually 2 or 3) were then to be implanted in BB's uterus. The procedure is expensive, and the success rate is variable. BB stated that she and her husband had decided to postpone discussing the impending procedure with their friends and family until pregnancy had been achieved. Both she and her husband, however, were emotionally prepared to become parents in 9 months.

Then BB reported that a complication had occurred during the procedure. After she had been readied to undergo implantation and was lying on the examination table, the tray containing 3 embryos was knocked over, and the embryos were destroyed. The doctor briefly apologized as the nurse mopped up the floor, and then everyone except BB left the room. She felt that she and her husband were somehow being punished by this failure; they had paid dearly, both in money and in emotional costs, to undergo the procedure. BB felt that the experience was too private and bizarre to share with anyone, and when she tried to talk about it with her husband, he was not receptive. She noted that since that event, she had often dreamed about babies, umbilical cords, and embryos.

She stated that she felt confused and that she was not sure what had happened; whether, in her words, she had "had a miscarriage, or an abortion, or nothing at all."

Diagnosis
Grief reaction

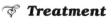 Treatment
- Counseling from a mental health provider.

- Practicing yoga 1 to 3 times weekly for stress reduction and relaxation (see Chapter 3).

- Completing a handwork project (see Chapter 5).

Follow Up
At her follow-up appointment 8 weeks later, BB reported that she was experiencing improved sleep, fewer intrusive thoughts, and an increased ability to concentrate. She had noted no episodes of chest pain or shortness of breath.

Discussion
In my opinion, BB's symptoms were a reaction to grief, and I advised her to define the experience as a type of miscarriage. The most prominent stages of grief are denial, anger, guilt, and acceptance. Each person experiences those stages for a different duration, although intense physical symptoms usually resolve 6 to 8 weeks after the loss occurred. Sharing grief with a friend or family member is the most powerful factor in recovery.

Failed infertility procedures are a significant loss for many women, and the grief of those patients should be acknowledged and honored. We as physicians often forget that even as technology advances, human emotions such as grief and disappointment remain unchanged. Many people in Western cultures avoid talking about death or loss, but that type of emotional sharing and bonding is essential to finding peace and moving forward.

Case 3. Flashbacks and Other Demons from the Past

CC, a 38-year-old woman, sought consultation at our clinic. She had stopped taking oral contraceptives 9 months earlier because she was concerned that the long-term use of synthetic hormones would increase her risk of breast cancer, which had afflicted several female family members. She said that she had been told by 2 physicians that the results of her blood tests, physical examination, and ultrasonography were within the normal range. Despite those assurances, she stated that she "didn't feel right."

CC's symptoms included decreased libido, irritability without cause, fatigue, headaches, feelings of despondency, and increased distractibility. She had difficulty sleeping and experienced food cravings, bloating, and unexplained aches and pains. She stated that she sometimes felt overwhelmed and out of control, which were new feelings for her.

At the time of her examination, CC had 2 children. She noted that as they grew older, she experienced more intrusive thoughts about her own childhood, which had been very traumatic. She was experiencing flashbacks and unpleasant thoughts almost every day. She also suffered from frequent nightmares, one of which she shared with me. CC was remorseful about the effects of her mood swings on her work and relationships. Consuming alcohol helped ease her symptoms, but she knew that substance abuse was not a long-term solution. She felt mortified after having recently eaten a half tube of raw chocolate chip cookie dough to placate her food cravings and irritability. She had taken dandelion root, black cohosh, kava kava, and St. John's wort to treat the symptoms described above, but those treatments were either ineffective or caused adverse effects.

At the time of her examination, CC was treating her headaches as needed with a combination tablet of acetaminophen, aspirin, and caffeine (Excedrin). She was taking acetaminophen plus diphenhydramine (Tylenol PM) at bedtime. She had suffered from childhood asthma and had undergone the removal of a benign breast tumor when she was in her 20s. She had begun to menstruate at the age of 14 years and had begun to use oral contraception (her preferred method of avoiding pregnancy) when she was 19 years of age. She had stopped taking oral contraceptives 9 months before her examination and was experiencing 28-day menstrual cycles.

CC's first pregnancy had occurred when she was 29 years of age. The vaginal delivery of an infant girl was routine, and she breastfed her daughter for 4 months. CC was 32 years of age when her son was born via a routine vaginal delivery. She breastfed her second child for 6 months.

CC's mother suffered from hypothyroidism, and the health status of her father was unknown. When CC's maternal grandmother was in her 40s and premenopausal, she suffered from breast cancer. CC's maternal aunt was postmenopausal and in her 50s when breast cancer was diagnosed.

When I examined CC, she was living with her husband and 2 children. She had been married for 10 years and worked part-time. She had a college education. CC had stopped exercising because of fatigue. She said that she had to nap during the evening and was too tired to cook. As a result, she and her family often consumed frozen dinners and fast food. She did not smoke, and she drank 3 to 5 alcoholic beverages per week.

The results of CC's physical examination were normal. Saliva testing revealed the following results:

Estradiol: Normal
Progesterone: Very low
Progesterone-estradiol ratio: Very low
Testosterone: Very low
Dehydroepiandrosterone sulfate (DHEAS): Normal
Cortisol: Morning - High
　　　　　Noon - Low
　　　　　Evening - High
　　　　　Bedtime – High

Diagnosis
Premenopause, deficiencies of progesterone and testosterone, posttraumatic stress disorder (PTSD), adrenal dysfunction

☞ Treatment
I prescribed the following therapies to address CC's hormone deficiencies and her PTSD:

- A topical bioidentical progesterone cream 40 mg/mL (0.5 mL to be applied to a thin-skinned area such as the inner arm or inner thigh once daily on days 1 to 10 of CC's menstrual cycle, then 1 mL to be applied once daily to a different thin-skinned site on cycle days 11 to 28) (see Chapter 6).

- Testosterone 4 mg in oil (1 oral capsule daily) (see Chapter 6).

- A calcium supplement containing vitamin D and magnesium.

- Referral to a therapist for treatment with eye movement desensitization and reprocessing (EMDR). EMDR therapy can eliminate or greatly decrease the emotional distress that is related to memories of traumatic events, even if they occurred years ago. In my opinion, EMDR can help victims of childhood sexual or physical abuse to reclaim the sense of self that was once violated and long silenced. During EMDR therapy, the patient recalls a past or present traumatic experience in brief episodes while performing a series of eye movements or focusing on an external stimulus such as auditory tones or tapping. After a rest period, the patient associates a positive thought with the memory of the unpleasant event.

- Decreased consumption of caffeine, refined foods, and sugars, all of which can exacerbate hormone imbalance.

- Increased consumption of protein, whole grains, and water.

- Consumption of broccoli, cauliflower, or cabbage (foods shown to be protective against breast cancer)[1] at least 3 times weekly.

- Eating meals prepared at home more frequently, which could be accomplished by planning menus in advance and enlisting help from family members or friends.

- Enrolling in a yoga class or following a home-based video program of yoga instruction 3 times weekly (see Chapter 3).

- Beginning a symptoms diary in which physical symptoms, feelings, and responses to stressful situations are recorded.

- Scheduling a Bio-Touch session once weekly (see Chapter 7).

☞ Cinematherapy
- *Parenthood*

- *Finding Nemo*

- *The Prince of Tides*

- *The Joy Luck Club*

☞ Suggested reading
Sanford LT. *Strong at the Broken Places: Overcoming the Trauma of Childhood Abuse.* New York, NY: Random House; 1990.

Bolen JS. Ring of Power: *The Abandoned Child, the Authoritarian Father, and the Disempowered Feminine: A Jungian Understanding of Wagner's Ring Cycle.* San Francisco, Calif: HarperSanFrancisco; 1992.

Wilson JL *Adrenal Fatigue: The 21st Century Stress Syndrome.* Petaluma, Calif: Smart Publications; 2001. Web site: www.adrenalfatigue.org.

☞ Internet resource
www.emdr.org — EMDR Institute, Inc - Information on eye movement desensitization and reprocessing (EMDR).

Follow Up
At her 8-week follow-up examination, CC had obtained relief from bloating and aches and pains. She stated that her quality of sleep and energy level had improved. She craved sugar less and had experienced fewer mood swings. She felt more in control in her relationships and roles and said that EMDR therapy was helpful in

reducing the frequency of intrusive thoughts and nightmares. The results of her physical examination and laboratory testing were normal, and her levels of cortisol were closer to normal values.

Discussion

CC's symptoms were caused by a profound lack of progesterone and testosterone (see Chapter 6). Because her symptoms were so severe, I recommended BHRT in addition to changes in diet and lifestyle. CC was concerned about the adverse effects and possible masculinization caused by testosterone supplementation, but I reassured her that our goal was to increase the level of that hormone to a normal physiologic range and not to oversupplement (which induces masculinization).

Before treatment was initiated, CC's cortisol profile was a concern, although an elevated evening value is common in women with children. The evening specimen for cortisol analysis is collected between 4:00 PM and 5:00 PM, a difficult time of day when small children are fussy, whiny, and irritable; pets are more active; family members arrive home from work; and the doorbell and telephone always seem to ring. I have found that restoring the balance of the sex steroid hormones in addition to implementing changes in diet and lifestyle changes can resolve imbalances in cortisol levels.

PTSD is common in women who revisit their girlhood as part of their midlife journey. Traumatic childhood experiences can affect health in adulthood. Research reveals an association between having been the victim of violence during childhood and the later development of adult-onset obesity, alcoholism, drug abuse, heart disease, and cancer, as well as dysregulation of the stress response caused by cortisol release.[2] A Swedish study showed that knowing whether a patient suffered violence or abuse during childhood is important in the diagnosis of common illnesses in women 40 to 50 years of age.[3] Although such findings are ominous, I have observed that many women overcome a tragic early life and enjoy good long-term health as adults.

References

1. Willet WC. Diet and breast cancer. *J Intern Med.* 2001;249(5):395-411.

2. Felitti VJ, Anda RF, Nordenberg D, et al. Relationship of childhood abuse and household dysfunction to many of the leading causes of death in adults. The Adverse Childhood Experiences (ACE) Study. *Am J Prev Med.* 1998;14(4):245-258.

3. Krantz G, Ostergren PO. The association between violence victimisation and common symptoms in Swedish women. *J Epidemiol Community Health.* 2000;54(11):815-821.

Case 4. Headaches and Hormones

DD, a 41-year-old woman, was concerned about her long-term use of oral contraceptives. She had used that form of contraception for 21 years but had recently discontinued its use. She reported symptoms of fluid retention; abdominal bloating; breast fullness and tenderness; irritability; hypersensitivity to grasses, pollens, and molds, which produced allergic rhinitis; and sleep disturbance. During the previous year she had gained 10 pounds, primarily in her abdomen, hips, and thighs. Her symptoms had gradually worsened over the prior 18 months. She reported that during the 3 years before her office visit, she had experienced 8 to 10 migraines per month.

DD's migraines were treated with either a combination of butalbital, acetaminophen, and caffeine (Esgic) as needed or with almotriptan malate (Axert). Her allergies were treated with loratadine (Claritin) as needed. She had undergone no prior surgeries. DD's menstrual periods occurred every 28 to 30 days. She had experienced 2 normal pregnancies with normal deliveries in her 20s. She had not breastfed either infant.

DD's mother was overweight and suffered from migraines and high blood pressure. Her father had diabetes, high blood pressure, heart disease, and a high cholesterol level. Her sister suffered from rheumatoid arthritis, and a maternal aunt had had breast cancer.

At the time of her visit, DD lived with her spouse. She worked part-time as a nurse and volunteered in her community. She was very close to her family members and often served as a problem solver and source of emotional support for them. She reported feeling frustrated when they did not follow her nursing advice or make good health choices. DD drank 3 glasses of wine per week. She did not smoke, and she followed an aerobic exercise program 4 to 5 times weekly. She ate a low-fat diet that included fresh fruits and vegetables.

DD's weight was normal for her height. Physical examination indicated mild fibrocystic changes in both breasts. Saliva testing revealed the following results:

> Estradiol: Normal
> Progesterone: Low
> Progesterone-estradiol ratio: Low
> Testosterone: Normal
> Dehydroepiandrosterone sulfate (DHEAS): Normal
> Cortisol: Morning - High
>   Noon - Normal
>   Evening - Normal
>   Bedtime - Normal

Diagnosis
Estrogen dominance, progesterone deficiency, migraine, adrenal dysfunction

☞ *Treatment*

To correct DD's hormone imbalances and prevent her migraines, I prescribed the following therapy:

- Bioidentical progesterone cream 40 mg/mL (0.5 mL to be applied to a thin-skinned area such as the inner arm or inner thigh on days 1 to 10 of her menstrual cycle, then 0.5 mL to be applied to a different thin-skinned area each morning and 1 mL to be likewise applied at bedtime on cycle days 11 to 28). I recommend that women who have migraines use topically applied hormones to prevent rapid fluctuations in hormone levels that can be caused by oral dosing (see Chapter 6).

- A calcium supplement containing vitamin D and magnesium.

- Decreasing the consumption of caffeine, refined foods, and sugars.

- Increasing the consumption of proteins, whole grains, and water.

- Practicing yoga 3 times weekly (see Chapter 3).

- Scheduling a Bio-Touch session once weekly and at the onset of migraine (see Chapter 7).

- Keeping a diary of symptoms.

- Completing a handwork project (see Chapter 5).

☞ *Cinematherapy*
- *Chocolat*

- *What's Cooking?*

☞ Suggested reading

Borysenko J. *Guilt Is the Teacher, Love Is the Lesson.* New York, NY: Warner Books, Inc; 1990.

Lee JR, Zava D, Hopkins H. *What Your Doctor May Not Tell You About Breast Cancer: How Hormone Balance Can Save Your Life.* New York, NY: Warner Books, Inc; 2002.

Forward S, Frazier D. *Emotional Blackmail: When the People in Your Life Use Fear, Obligation, and Guilt to Manipulate You.* New York, NY: HarperCollins Publishers, 1997.

Follow Up

At her 8-week follow-up appointment, DD reported a weight loss of 3 pounds. She was practicing yoga at least 3 times each week. Her symptom diary revealed that she was experiencing fewer headaches (now 4 to 5 per month) that were less intense. The quality of her sleep had improved, she had more energy, and her mood was better in general, although she reported a negative mood and bloating in the late second half of her menstrual cycle.

☞ *Treatment Modification*

- Bioidentical progesterone cream 40 mg/mL (1 mL to be applied to the skin as before at bedtime on days 1 to 10 of her menstrual cycle, then 1 mL to be applied to a different thin-skinned area in the morning and at bedtime from cycle day 11 until the start of menstruation).

- Repeat saliva testing before the next office visit.

Secondary Follow Up

After having followed the modified treatment regimen for 16 weeks, DD reported a weight loss of 5 pounds. She had experienced only 2 minor headaches during the month before her second follow-up visit. She stated that the symptoms that usually occurred during the last half of her menstrual cycle had diminished in severity. Saliva testing revealed that all hormone values were within the normal range.

Discussion

Migraines are diagnosed in twice as many women as men, and hormone-related migraines affect about 12 million women in the United States.[1] During the transition to menopause, fluctuating estrogen and progesterone levels may be associated with the frequency of migraines and seizure disorders. The balance of estrogen and progesterone affects the levels of substances in the brain that induce migraines and seizures. I have observed that some patients experience new-onset migraines in their premenopausal years, when the level of estrogen is high relative to that of progesterone. Evidence shows that girls have an increased incidence of seizures during their early pubertal years, a time at which the level of estrogen is also high relative to that of progesterone.[2] Treatment with bioidentical progesterone, which can restore a normal estradiol-progesterone ratio, in addition to changes in diet and lifestyle, can be helpful in the management of migraines and seizure disorders.

References

1. DeMasi MA. Hormonally associated migraine. *The Female Patient.* 2004;29(7):30-36.

2. Jette N, Morrell MJ. Sex-steroid hormones in women with epilepsy. *The Female Patient.* 2004;29(7):23-29.

Case 5. Too Much to Do, Too Little Time

EE, a 41-year-old female patient, complained of a weight gain of 10 pounds over the prior 6 months, a craving for sugar, mood swings, night sweats, aches and pains, premenstrual and menstrual migraines, fatigue, despondent mood, and dry hair and skin. For the past 3 years, she had suffered from migraines. Her prior physician had told her that "Everything is normal."

EE had been treating her headaches with a combination of aspirin, acetaminophen, and caffeine (Excedrin) as needed. When she was in her 20s, she had experienced 2 normal pregnancies that culminated in normal deliveries. Her menstrual periods occurred every 28 days, and she was not sexually active. EE had undergone no prior surgeries. Her mother had had diabetes, her father was healthy, and her maternal grandmother had suffered from diabetes and breast cancer.

At the time of her appointment, EE was the divorced mother of 2 teenagers. She worked full-time in a management position. She stated that she did not exercise, she consumed 2 to 3 alcoholic beverages per month, and she did not smoke. She described her choice of food as "the Soccer Mom Diet," which is common fare when children are too young to drive themselves to their many activities and their mother eats on the go while shuttling them to their classes, commitments, practices, and events. She also stated that her children were overweight.

EE reported that she usually skipped breakfast so that she could sleep longer in the morning. She often ate food from a vending machine or fast food for lunch. The father of EE's children lived in another state and did not send child support. She referred to occasional conflicts with her adolescent children.

EE was obese. Physical examination revealed an enlarged thyroid, fibrocystic changes in both breasts, coolness of the hands and feet, and coarse, dry hair and skin. Her score on the Beck Depression Inventory indicated mild depression. Serum and saliva testing revealed the following values:

Serum testing (range)
Thyroid hormones: Thyroid-stimulating hormone (TSH) - High
Free triiodothyronine (T_3) and free levothyroxine (T_4) - Low

Saliva testing (range)
Estradiol: Normal
Progesterone: Low
Progesterone-estradiol ratio: Normal
Testosterone: Low
Dehydroepiandrosterone sulfate (DHEAS): Normal
Cortisol: Morning - High
Bedtime - Low

Diagnosis
Estrogen dominance, progesterone deficiency, hypothyroidism, mild depression, adrenal dysfunction

☞ Treatment
I prescribed the following regimen for EE:

- A bioidentical progesterone cream 30 mg/mL (0.5 mL to be applied to a thin-skinned area such as the inner thigh or inner arm on days 1 to 10 of her menstrual cycle, then 0.5 mL to be applied to a different thin-skinned area in the morning and 1 mL to be applied in the evening from cycle day 11 until the start of menstruation) (see Chapter 6).

- Testosterone 4 mg in oil (1 capsule daily) (see Chapter 6).

- Thyroid tablets, USP, (Armour thyroid) 15 mg (1 tablet each morning for 3 weeks, then 2 tablets [a total of 30 mg] each morning as a maintenance dosage) (see Chapter 6).

- Planning weekly menus on Saturday and Sunday and involving her children in meal planning and preparation. Although this type of advance planning might seem difficult, it is a tremendous timesaver and prevents reliance on fast food for a quick meal.

- Eating a homecooked evening meal 3 times weekly (goal, eating 5 family meals at home weekly). Research from Harvard University showed that in children 9 to 14 years of age, eating at home was associated with better nutrition; the increased consumption of fruits, vegetables, and fiber; and the decreased consumption of soda, sugar, and saturated fats.[1] Other research indicates that in the evaluation of more than 500 adolescents, those who ate a family meal at home at least 5 days per week demonstrated better academic performance, greater self-esteem, better choices in peer relationships, less likelihood of illicit drug use, and a lower incidence of depression than did teenagers who ate a meal at home 3 times weekly or less.[2] I have recently become concerned about families in my care who have completely stopped grocery shopping and cooking at home and eat out instead. Those patients have stated that eating out is convenient and that the cost of having the family dinner at an all-you-can eat buffet is about the same as or less than that of eating at home. Although eating primarily in restaurants may seem to be time-efficient and economical, I believe that families who do so pay a great price in potential adverse health-related effects. Children are worth the effort of preparing a home-cooked meal, the benefits of which are not limited to nutrition.

- Taking a nutritionally balanced lunch to work.

- Eating a nutritionally balanced breakfast each day, perhaps in the car while driving her children to school.

- Increasing water intake and keeping an ice chest containing bottled water and low-fat snacks in the car to answer the perpetual "I'm hungry, I'm thirsty" cry.

- Decreasing caffeine consumption to 2 caffeine-containing beverages per day.

- Practicing yoga 1 to 3 times weekly (see Chapter 3).

- Exercising while waiting for her the children, perhaps by walking around the soccer field or parking lot or climbing stairs or bleachers rather than sitting in the car.

- Restricting computer leisure time and the viewing of television and videos to less than 2 hours daily.

- Keeping a diary of symptoms.

- Scheduling a Bio-Touch session once weekly (see Chapter 7).

- Beginning a handwork project that could be completed while waiting at meetings, events, and her children's practices. By engaging in handwork, EE would be less likely to eat when bored. She would also benefit from the positive neurologic and cardiovascular benefits of handwork (see Chapter 5).

☞ Cinematherapy
- *Freaky Friday*

- *Super Size Me*

☞ Suggested reading
Bassoff E. *Mothers and Daughters: Loving and Letting Go.* New York, NY: New American Library; 1988.

Pipher MB. *Reviving Ophelia: Saving the Selves of Adolescent Girls.* New York, NY: Ballantine Books; 2001.

Kabat-Zinn M, Kabat-Zinn J. *Everyday Blessings: The Inner Work of Mindful Parenting.* New York, NY: Hyperion; 1997.

Katzen M. *The New Enchanted Broccoli Forest.* Berkeley, Calif: Ten Speed Press; 2000.

Katzen M. *Mollie Katzen's Sunlight Cafe.* New York, NY: Hyperion; 2002.

Katzen M. *The New Moosewood Cookbook.* Berkeley, Calif: Ten Speed Press, 2000.

Cooking Light magazine — Healthy, simple, family-friendly recipes.

Schlosser E. *Fast Food Nation: The Dark Side of the All-American Meal.* Boston, Mass: Houghton Mifflin; 2001.

Follow Up
At her 12-week follow-up appointment, EE had lost 15 pounds. She reported having fewer and less severe headaches, a decrease in her craving for sugar, and fewer night sweats. Her depressed mood had lifted, but she still noted periodic midday fatigue and "fuzzy thinking." Repeat serum and saliva testing revealed that all sex-steroid values previously evaluated had improved and that her levels of T_3 and T_4 were slightly low.

☞ Treatment Modification
- Addition of compounded T_3 7.5 mcg (1 capsule at midday, a dosage that could be increased to twice daily if needed) to relieve midday fatigue and cognitive sluggishness. Some patients require

supplementation with both T_3 and T_4 to relieve the symptoms of hypothyroidism.[3]

Secondary Follow Up

At her 24-week follow-up appointment, EE reported that her energy level had increased and that she was practicing yoga or participating in an aerobic exercise program 4 to 5 times weekly. Her weight was in the normal range for her height. Repeat serum and saliva testing revealed that all hormone values previously evaluated were within the normal range. EE stated that her children's health status had also improved because beneficial changes in diet and lifestyle had been made as a family.

Discussion

Like many women, EE had developed a pattern of neglecting her own emotional and physical health. As a single mother of 2 teenagers, she was highly stressed and focused her efforts on meeting financial obligations and being both mother and father to her children. A combination of the Soccer Mom Diet and many hours of inactivity (sitting at her desk all day, sitting in her car or in a chair during her children's afterschool activities, and then sitting on the couch in the evening because she was exhausted) worsened EE's hormone imbalance and hypothyroidism. As her teenagers began their quest for independence, her relationship with them changed to conflict instead of mutual emotional support and comfort. Understanding her need for self-care and thinking of herself as an individual apart from her professional and parental roles were important in EE's treatment and attainment of a better level of health.

References

1. Gillman MW, Rifas-Shiman SL, Frazier AL, et al. Family dinner and diet quality among older children and adolescents. *Arch Fam Med.* 2000;9(3):235-240.

2. Bowden BS, Zeisz JM. Supper's on! Adolescent adjustment and frequency of family mealtimes. Paper presented at: 105th Annual Convention of the American Psychological Association; August 16, 1997; Chicago, Ill.

3. Bunevicius R, Kazanavicius G, Zalinkevicius R, Prange AJ Jr. Effects of thyroxine as compared with thyroxine plus triiodothyronine in patients with hypothyroidism. *N Engl J Med.* 1999;340(6):424-429.

Case 6. Ignoring Symptoms, Delaying Care

FF, a 41-year-old female patient, complained about a cough of 3 months' duration. She stated that she had been treating herself with antibiotics obtained from friends but that the cough had not gone away. Because she did not have insurance and was in very difficult social circumstances, she had not been able to consult a physician. During the 2 months before her visit, she had lost 10 pounds and her appetite had decreased, but she attributed those symptoms to having experienced recent stress.

At the time of her appointment, the only medication used by FF was an over-the-counter cough medication that she took as needed. She had had no prior illnesses and had undergone a tubal ligation when she was in her 30s after having experienced 2 normal pregnancies with normal deliveries. Her menstrual periods occurred every 28 to 30 days, and she was not sexually active.

FF had been divorced twice. A few months before her appointment, she had ended an abusive relationship suddenly and had left her shared residence with only the clothes that she was wearing. She then lived in her car for a few weeks while her 2 adolescent children stayed with friends. A few weeks later, a female coworker invited FF to stay in her home for a few weeks until she could save enough money to rent an apartment.

FF worked as a nurse. She smoked 2 to 3 packs of cigarettes per day and had been smoking since she was 14 years old. She did not drink alcohol, and she stated that her diet was poor because of the upheaval in her living situation.

Physical examination revealed that FF was underweight for her height. Her breath sounds were abnormal, as were the results of her lung examinationl: Radiographs revealed large masses consistent with lung cancer. FF underwent the biopsy of those masses to confirm the suspected diagnosis.

Diagnosis
Lung cancer

☞ Treatment
Referral to an oncologist and to a social worker.

Follow Up
By the time of diagnosis, FF's lung cancer had metastasized to her liver and brain. Her first concern after she was informed of her prognosis was for the well-being of her children. A team of nurses, social workers, doctors, friends, and teachers worked together to find a secure environment for them. FF's medical condition worsened just before Christmas, and the hospital staff created a special holiday celebration for FF and her children in her hospital room. FF did not respond to treatment for her cancer and made the decision to enter hospice. She died a few months after diagnosis.

Discussion
Cancer of the lung is the leading cause of death from cancer in US men and women.[1] In the United States, more people die of lung cancer each year than from breast cancer, prostate cancer, and colon cancer combined.[1]

Research has shown that women with some types of lung cancer respond more favorably to surgery and chemotherapy than do men with that same type of cancer.[2] Other studies have shown that women who smoke may be more likely to develop lung cancer at a younger age.[3]

Gender, gene expression, and immune factors are also thought to affect the development of lung cancer and the patient's response to treatment.[1-3] Because they need a flexible work schedule or part-time employment, many women who are full-time caregivers must accept employment without medical benefits. Early diagnosis may improve the length of survival of any patient with cancer, but like FF, many women with few social and financial resources do not seek medical care. Instead, they use the little money they have to meet their children's needs. Uninsured women carry a large burden of illness in the United States. Unfortunately, screening for many serious diseases and much-needed medical care are priced beyond their grasp. Government agencies, physicians, employers, and community organizations must to work together to make health care more accessible for women like FF.

References

1. American Cancer Society Web site. Available at: www.cancer.org. Accessed June 18, 2004.

2. Dresler CM, Fratelli C, Babb J, Everley L, Evans AA, Clapper ML. Gender differences in genetic susceptibility for lung cancer. *Lung Cancer.* 2000;30(3): 153-160.

3. Radzikowska E, Glaz P, Roszkowski K. Lung cancer in women: age, smoking, histology, performance status, stage, initial treatment and survival. Population-based study of 20 561 cases. *Ann Oncol.* 2002;13(7): 1087-1093.

Case 7. The Blues of the Stay-At-Home Mom

GG, a 41-year-old stay-at-home mother, complained of a variety of symptoms: hot flashes that had begun after she underwent hysterectomy, the removal of both ovaries, and bladder suspension 4 years earlier; night sweats;

mood swings that ranged from hyperirritability to apathy; hypersomnia (she went to bed from the time that her children left for school until they returned home); low energy; headaches; decreased libido; bloating; cognitive slowing; a craving for sugar; and weight gain (she reported that she weighed more than when she had been pregnant). GG was unable to name any hobbies or experiences that she found pleasurable.

At the time of her appointment, GG was being treated with oral estradiol (Estrace) 2 mg daily to relieve menopausal symptoms and omeprazole (Prilosec) as needed for the treatment of gastroesophageal reflux. She had received venlafaxine hydrochloride (Effexor) for last 3 years as treatment for depression. GG also suffered from migraines and irritable bowel syndrome. She had experienced 5 normal pregnancies, each of which culminated in the delivery of a healthy infant. Three of those 5 deliveries were accomplished by cesarean section.

GG's father had died of cancer. Her mother had thyroid disease, her maternal grandmother suffered from heart disease, and her sister was addicted to illicit drugs. GG described herself as a "stay-at-home" mom. She lived with her spouse and 4 of her children, who ranged in age from 6 to 15 years. She prepared all of her family's mcals at home.

GG had a college education. She did not smoke or drink alcohol. She stated that she did not exercise but instead spent her leisure time attending to her children's needs and activities. She had been active as a volunteer in her church, but there had been a recent conflict among the members of the congregation and she had recently stopped attending services and performing volunteer work there.

GG was obese. Physical examination revealed thinning scalp hair, a slightly enlarged thyroid, and coarse, dry hair and skin. Her score on the Zung Self-Rating Depression Scale was classified as moderate. Serum and saliva testing revealed the following results:

Serum testing (range)
> Thyroid hormones: Normal

Saliva testing (range)
> Estradiol: Normal
> Progesterone: Low
> Progesterone-estradiol ratio: Low
> Testosterone: Normal
> Dehydroepiandrosterone sulfate (DHEAS): Normal
> Cortisol: Morning - Low
> > Noon - Normal
> > Evening - High
> > Bedtime – Low

Diagnosis

Estrogen dominance, progesterone deficiency, depression, adrenal dysfunction, obesity, migraines, irritable bowel syndrome

☞ Treatment

- Gradually decrease and then eliminate the use of venlafaxine hydrochloride (Effexor).

- Begin treatment with bupropion hydrochloride (Wellbutrin), an antidepressant that increases dopamine activity.

- A combination of bioidentical hormones (80% estriol and 20% estradiol [Bi-Est] 0.375 mg/mL plus progesterone 40 mg/mL) in a cream (1 mL to be applied to a thin-skinned area such as the inner thigh or inner arm at bedtime) (see Chapter 6).

- Thyroid tablets, USP (Armour thyroid) 15 mg (1 tablet in the morning) (see Chapter 6).

- A calcium supplement plus vitamins E, B complex, and C.

- Increase the daily intake of protein and water.

- Practice yoga 1 to 3 times weekly (see Chapter 3).

- Keep a diary of symptoms.

- Schedule a Bio-Touch session once weekly (see Chapter 7).

- Participate in a local or online support group for stay-at-home mothers.

☞ Cinematherapy
- *The Apostle*

- *Tender Mercies*

☞ Suggested reading
Crittenden D. *Amanda.bright@home*. New York, NY: Warner Books; 2003.

Wilson JL. *Adrenal Fatigue: The 21st Century Stress Syndrome* Petaluma, Calif: Smart Publications; 2001. Web site: www.adrenalfatigue.org.

Northrup C. *The Wisdom of Menopause: Creating Physical and Emotional Health and Healing During the Change*. New York, NY: Bantam Books; 2001.

Follow Up
At her 8-week follow-up appointment, GG said that she had experienced no adverse effects from treatment with bioidentical hormone replacement therapy or bupropion

hydrochloride (Wellbutrin). She reported improved mood, fewer food cravings, better concentration, and greater energy. She had lost 7 pounds and was interacting more with her husband and children instead of withdrawing from them.

Discussion

GG's symptoms (the loss of the ability to feel pleasure [anhedonia], food cravings, decreased libido, a reduced ability to achieve orgasm, and decreased concentration) were related to imbalances of hormones and neurotransmitters. The prolonged chronic use of an antidepressant that blocks serotonin uptake may, over time, create undesirable effects such as apathy, weight gain, and sexual dysfunction. Those effects are thought to be related to a decrease in dopamine activity, an important neurotransmitter. The use of the antidepressant bupropion hydrochloride (Wellbutrin), which increases dopamine activity, alleviated those symptoms in GG.

The emotional needs of stay-at-home mothers are often forgotten. It is as if, by choosing to work in the home, those women lose their rights. Talking about stress and frustration is helpful in diffusing tension, but stay-at-home women often feel isolated and hesitate to share their dilemmas or to complain. Our society often does not recognize the tremendous sacrifice and service that these women contribute. I believe that their role in providing secure attachments for their children, homecooked and healthful nutrition, and daily emotional support should be greatly valued and not scorned. I have found that my role as a mother and as what Virginia Woolf termed "the angel of the house" has been much more difficult for me emotionally and physically than my role as a physician.

Case 8. Surviving the Greatest Loss of All

HH, a 42-year-old woman, complained of night sweats, hyperirritability, decreased libido, thinning hair, fatigue, food cravings, and depressed mood. Those symptoms had been present for more than a year. She reported a weight gain of 20 pounds over the past 12 months. To treat symptoms, her former primary care physician had suggested injections of either synthetic estrogen or olanzapine (Zyprexa), which is an antipsychotic medication. HH was reluctant to receive injections of a synthetic hormone, but she agreed to olanzapine therapy because she was desperate to obtain symptom relief. However, treatment-related adverse effects caused her to stop therapy with that drug.

Two years before her office visit, HH had undergone a vaginal hysterectomy and the removal of her left ovary. She had experienced 2 normal pregnancies with normal deliveries when she was in her 20s. Her mother had suffered from heart disease, and her father had died of congestive heart failure. Her sister, who was obese, was afflicted with diabetes and heart disease.

At the time of her visit, HH lived with her spouse and 1 of her 2 children. Her other child had died in an accident 2 years earlier. HH worked full time in management. She drank 2 glasses of wine per week and did not smoke. She did not exercise and admitted that her diet was poor.

Physical examination showed that HH was obese and that her scalp hair was thinning. Serum and saliva testing revealed the following results:

Serum testing (range)
> Thyroid hormones: Normal

Saliva testing (range)
Estradiol: Normal
Progesterone: Low
Progesterone-estradiol ratio: Low
Testosterone: Normal
Dehydroepiandrosterone (DHEAS): Normal
Cortisol: Morning - High
Noon - Normal
Evening - High
Bedtime - High

HH's score on a standardized scale that measures stress levels was very high, as was her score on the Beck Depression Inventory, an evaluation of clinical depression.

Diagnosis
Clinical depression, estrogen dominance, progesterone deficiency, adrenal dysfunction

☞ Treatment
- Bioidentical progesterone cream 30 mg/mL (1 mL to be applied to a thin-skinned area such as the inner thigh or inner arm at bedtime) (see Chapter 6).

- Discontinuing treatment with Zyprexa, which produced adverse effects.

- Beginning therapy with bupropion (Wellbutrin) to treat depression.

- Creating weekly menus that included several homecooked meals.

- Consulting a psychotherapist.

- Preparing lunches to take to work as opposed to selecting food from vending machines or a convenience store.

- Decreasing the consumption of caffeine, refined foods, and sugar.

- Increasing the consumption of protein, whole grains, and water.

- Practicing yoga 3 times weekly in addition to following instruction on the *Yoga at Your Desk* CD (Palos Verdes Estates, Calif: VN Industries, Inc; 2001) (see Chapter 3).

- Connecting with The Compassionate Friends, a support group designed for parents who have experienced the trauma of a child's death (see the Internet resources listed below).

- Completing a handwork project (see Chapter 5).

☞ *Cinematherapy*
- *What Dreams May Come*

- *The Dollmaker*

☞ *Suggested reading*
Cobb N. *In Lieu of Flowers: A Conversation for the Living.* New York, NY: Pantheon Books; 2000.

Follow Up

At her 8-week follow-up visit, HH reported a weight loss of 7 pounds. She noted that her mood was more even, and she had observed an improvement in her hair and skin. She was no longer experiencing night sweats, and she had more energy. She had attended The Compassionate Friends support group and had found it beneficial.

Discussion

HH suffered from a hormone imbalance as well as depression. In women with mild depression, bioidentical hormone replacement therapy (BHRT) often exerts a mood-stabilizing effect, and the need for antidepressant therapy is obviated. If the depression is severe, however, treatment with an antidepressant is often needed in addition to psychotherapy.

Many drug therapies for treating clinical depression are now available. Because HH was concerned about weight gain and decreased libido, I felt that Wellbutrin, which causes fewer adverse effects of that type, would be the best choice for her treatment. This case also illustrates the importance of the "test-and-treat" approach versus the "guess-and-treat" approach in treating women (see Chapter 6). HH's prior physician had recommended estrogen injections as 1 of 2 therapeutic options, but testing revealed that HH's estrogen level was in the normal range. HH had also suffered the death of a child, which is designated as the greatest possible stressor on most stress-assessment scales. At the conclusion of this case report, 2 poems written by a parent whose child died of sudden cardiac death are featured. Those heartfelt expressions of loss speak directly to all parents who have experienced a similar tragedy.

In my clinical experience, grieving parents benefit from talking with others who have endured a similar trauma. Support groups dedicated to that purpose, such as The Compassionate Friends, meet in many cities.

Internet resource:

www.compassionatefriends.org/ - A support group for those who have experienced the death of a child.

Poems on the Loss of a Child

The Heart
D.R. Balusek

They talk about the strength of one's heart,
How it can handle happiness, stress, love, and when a
love one departs.
A cycle of everyday life brings different people in,
Only a special few become true friends.

Our capacity to love is vast for friends and family,
But when one dies, the pain is beyond belief.
So if walking builds the muscle of the heart,
How long does one walk to keep sadness from tearing it
apart?

Never Coming Back
D.R. Balusek

I would sit by his bed when he was three,
Just to watch my little boy sleep.
He had a face of serenity, a smile of total peace,
He looked like the angel that he came to be.

I would always kiss his forehead right before I left,
If I had known the kiss in June would have been the last,
I would have done it again.
He had become stronger and his hug was so tight,
I did not know that hug would have to last the rest of my
life.

I would have extended my visit just to share more time,
To watch *Star Trek*, listen to music, and hear what was
on his mind.
Who do I ask when I hear a new song or read about an
unknown group?
We had special conversations and there will never be
anyone new.

As a child he would say "gakees" in order to see,
The word was "murk" when he was thirsty.
His smile would light a room and everyone would know
That he was the poster child, for he told them so.

Now when I am in a crowd, I have never felt so alone.
The phone will never ring with his special tone.
The foundation of my future is forever cracked,
For the son I love so much is never coming back.

Case 9. The Decision to Say Goodbye

VV, a woman in her early 40s, had been my patient for some time. She suffered from severe multiple sclerosis and was totally dependent on her husband, who provided care for all her physical needs. She could not walk, feed herself, or control her bowels or bladder. She was unable to speak but could make some guttural noises. Although she was unable to express her thoughts, her eyes conveyed intelligence and awareness. Her husband had supported her physically and emotionally from the moment of diagnosis and throughout her physical deterioration, from her use of a cane to her reliance on a wheelchair to her confinement in a hospital bed. He lovingly cared for her, and I remember how impressed I was with the excellent condition of her skin.

Shortly after the birth of her first grandchild and about 12 years after VV's multiple sclerosis had been diagnosed, she began to lose weight. Physical examination and laboratory testing indicated no cause for her weight loss or other significant changes in her health. VV's husband stated that she was not eating and that she drank very little. After a lengthy discussion, it was decided that VV should be referred to a specialist for placement of a feeding tube. Shortly before her appointment for that procedure, VV's husband requested to see me. He was very upset. He believed that his wife was refusing to eat or drink because she was ready to die. He remembered VV's having said that she wanted to live long enough to see the birth of her first grandchild, and he had been reflecting on that conversation. He said that he had found the courage to ask her if she was ready to die, and he felt that her answer was affirmative. He knew that a feeding tube would prolong her survival, and he couldn't imagine life without her. He also felt that he was being selfish in asking her to live with the discomfort and severe limitations imposed by her debilitating illness. We talked and cried, and he reminisced about their marriage and VV's illness. At the end of the visit, he asked me to cancel the appointment with the specialist and instead to call a hospice center so that he could arrange for his wife to receive end-of-life care. VV died peacefully and at home less than 1 month later.

Discussion

Discussing end-of-life care can be difficult, but the options of writing a living will and communicating wishes about hospice care, organ donation, and funeral arrangements greatly assist grieving family members or friends. Marriage and family relationships of deep love, commitment, and emotional maturity, like the relationship that VV and her husband shared, can make the transition from life to death more gentle. VV's husband was attentive to her wishes even though she could not verbally state her intention, and he honored her request.

Case 10. Too Tired for Sex

JJ, a 44-year-old female patient, expressed concerns about her hormone status. She complained of decreased libido, aches and pains, fatigue, a craving for sugar, an increase in pigmented patches on her face, and irritability (especially during the second half of her menstrual cycle). Because her menstrual periods occurred regularly every

28 to 30 days, her former physician had deduced that her symptoms were not related to a hormone imbalance.

JJ took a glucosamine chondroitin supplement and a multivitamin daily. She had undergone no prior surgery. She had experienced 3 normal pregnancies, each of which culminated in a normal delivery. After her last pregnancy, she had experienced postpartum depression that was treated with fluoxetine (Prozac). Her mother, who was in her 80s, suffered from dementia, and her father, who was also in his 80s, had high blood pressure. Her siblings were in good health.

At the time of her evaluation, JJ was living with her husband and 3 children. She was the caregiver for her parents, who lived nearby, and she worked part-time in health care. She reported that her stress level was high and that she felt as if she were always reacting to the demands of work, home, her children, or her elderly parents. She stated that she had a 23-day menstrual cycle. JJ's weight was normal for her height. She exercised by walking, ate a low-fat diet, and denied alcohol or tobacco use. Serum and saliva testing revealed the following results:

Serum testing (range)
　　Thyroid hormones: Normal

Saliva testing (range)
　　Estradiol: Normal
　　Progesterone: Low
　　Progesterone-estradiol ratio: Low
　　Testosterone: Normal
　　Cortisol: Morning - High
　　　　　　Noon - Normal
　　　　　　Evening - High
　　　　　　Bedtime – Normal

Diagnosis
Adrenal dysfunction, estrogen dominance, progesterone deficiency, female sexual arousal disorder

❧ Treatment
Because JJ preferred oral dosing, I prescribed the following regimen:

- Bioidentical progesterone extended-release 300-mg tablets (1 tablet to be taken at bedtime on days 1 to 6 of her menstrual cycle, then 1 tablet 2 to 4 times a daily [with at least 3 to 4 hours between doses] on cycle days 7 to 23) (see Chapter 6).

- Practicing yoga 1 to 3 times weekly (see Chapter 3).

- Keeping a diary of symptoms.

- Completing a handwork project (see Chapter 5).

- Scheduling a Bio-Touch session once weekly (see Chapter 7).

❧ Cinematherapy
- *The Preacher's Wife*

- *Michael*

❧ Suggested reading
Mayer A. *How To Stay Lovers While Raising Your Children*. Los Angeles, Calif: Price Stern Sloan; 1990.

Lee V. *Soulful Sex: Opening Your Heart, Body & Spirit to Lifelong Passion*. Berkeley, Calif: Conari Press; 1996.

Louden J. *The Couple's Comfort Book: A Creative Guide for Renewing Passion, Pleasure & Commitment*. New York, NY: HarperSanFrancisco; 1994.

Holstein LL. *How to Have Magnificent Sex: The 7 Dimensions of a Vital Sexual Connection*. New York, NY: Harmony Books; 2001.

Follow Up

At her 8-week follow-up appointment, JJ reported that treatment with progesterone in the prescribed dosage 3 times daily was most effective for her in the second half of her menstrual cycle. She felt better overall but stated that her libido had increased only slightly. She noted that a weekend away from home enabled her to relax, but when she returned to her daily environment she was highly stressed and her receptivity to sexual activity decreased.

Secondary Diagnosis

Female sexual arousal disorder

☞ Treatment Modification

- Compounded sildenafil (Viagra) 2% cream with optional flavoring, such as chocolate or pina colada, to be used as needed (a pea-size amount was to be placed on the clitoral area 20 to 30 minutes before sexual activity). An increase in the blood flow to the genitals is thought to trigger sexual responsiveness. I have found that about 40% of women who complain of diminished libido benefit to some degree from this treatment, but others find it ineffective or experience unpleasant sensations when the cream is applied. Those differences in the response to treatment may be due to the variability and complexity of female sexual arousal and response patterns.

Discussion

In families today, it is easy for parents to become so absorbed in problems with their children, job, finances, or house maintenance and with the care of aging parents that they forget their passion for each other. As couples mature and their relationship extends over decades, adaptations and changes in the bedroom and the living room are necessary to sustain a vibrant, mutually enjoyable intimate relationship. I have found that the "Weekend of Joy" exercise in the book *Soulful Sex: Opening Your Heart, Body & Spirit to Lifelong Passion* (see "Suggested reading") is especially beneficial for couples in circumstances similar to those described by JJ. That exercise involves a 36-hour respite from family and work demands during which the couple focus solely on each other. The exercise costs very little; the biggest obstacle is making arrangements for the care of children, pets, and aging parents. My clinical experience has shown, however, that it is well worth the effort, because the Weekend of Joy helps couples to reclaim and enrich their intimacy.

Case 11. Bad Genes? Overriding the Odds for Illness

KK, a 48-year-old woman, had been concerned about changes in her health. During the prior year, she had experienced irregular menstrual periods, fluid retention, abdominal bloating, cravings for sugar, night sweats, dry hair and skin, fatigue, a decreased ability to concentrate, sleep disturbances, and a weight gain of 30 pounds in her waist and abdomen. She was offered treatment with conjugated estrogens plus medroxyprogesterone acetate (Prempro) or citalopram (Celexa) by her primary care provider but refused both treatments.

Before she sought evaluation at our clinic, KK had treated her symptoms of fatigue by taking an over-the-counter supplement of dehydroepiandrosterone (DHEA). She had experienced no prior illnesses and had undergone no surgeries. When she was in her 20s, she had experienced 2 normal pregnancies, each of which culminated in a normal delivery. She did not breastfeed either infant. KK's mother died of gastrointestinal cancer, and her father, who had had diabetes, died of a heart attack. Her maternal grandmother had suffered a stroke but died of a heart attack.

At the time of her examination, KK was living with her husband, with whom she owned a small business. She denied alcohol and tobacco use but reported a diet high in fast food, fat, and sugar. She stated that she was "too tired to cook or exercise." KK was obese, and her blood pressure was slightly high. Physical examination revealed fibrocystic changes in her breasts. Serum and saliva testing revealed the following results:

Serum testing (range)
    Fasting glucose: High normal
    Fasting insulin: High
    High-density lipoprotein cholesterol (HDL): Low
    Total cholesterol: Normal
    Triglycerides: High
    Low-density lipoprotein cholesterol (LDL): Normal
    Thyroid hormones: Normal

Saliva testing (range)
    Estradiol: Normal
    Progesterone: Low
    Progesterone-estradiol ratio: Low
    Testosterone: High
    Dehydroepiandrosterone sulfate (DHEAS): High
    Cortisol: Morning - Normal
             Noon - Normal
             Evening - Normal
             Bedtime - High

Diagnosis
Metabolic syndrome, hormone imbalance, adrenal dysfunction, obesity

☞ *Treatment*

- Bioidentical progesterone cream 30 mg/mL (1 mL to be applied to a thin-skinned area such as the inner thigh or inner arm on days 1 to 10 of KK's menstrual cycle, then 1 mL to be applied to a different thin-skinned site in the morning and at bedtime from cycle day 11 until the start of menstruation) (see Chapter 6).

- Terminating treatment with over-the-counter DHEA.

- A daily supplement containing calcium, vitamin D, and magnesium.

- A daily multivitamin containing vitamins B, E, and C.

- A supplement containing chromium picolinate (400 mcg 3 times daily).

- Omega-3 fish oil, which improves cholesterol levels, lowers blood pressure, and prevents cardiovascular disease[1] (3 g daily in capsule form).

- Guggul extract (the dosage of which varies according to each patient's needs) to improve the levels of triglycerides and cholesterol and to enhance the effect of thyroid hormone activity at the cellular level.[2,3]

- Coenzyme Q_{10} for cardiovascular protection.[4,5]

- Consuming more foods that have a low glycemic index (the rate at which foods are converted into sugar and absorbed into the bloodstream). For example, the glycemic index of sugared carbonated soft drinks is very high, but that of vegetables and whole grains is low.

- Restricting fast-food consumption and following the Mediterranean diet as a model.[6] More information about the Mediterranean diet can be found in the Internet resource section.

- Practicing yoga 1 to 3 times weekly (see Chapter 3).

- Beginning a handwork project (see Chapter 5).

- Keeping a diary of symptoms and food consumed.

- Scheduling a Bio-Touch session once weekly (see Chapter 7).

☞ Suggested reading

Challem J, Berkson B, Smith MD. *Syndrome X: The Complete Nutritional Program to Prevent and Reverse Insulin Resistance.* New York, NY: Wiley; 2000.

Wilson JL. *Adrenal Fatigue: The 21st Century Stress Syndrome.* Petaluma, Calif: Smart Publications; 2001. Web site: www.adrenalfatigue.org.

☞ Internet resource

www.oldwayspt.org — A link to information about the Mediterranean diet.

Follow Up

At her 16-week follow-up examination, KK reported that she felt well and that her mood, energy level, and clarity of thought had improved since her prior visit. She had made the recommended lifestyle and nutritional changes. Her blood pressure and all prior abnormal laboratory testing values were within the normal range, and she had lost 20 pounds. She was experiencing less breast tenderness and bloating and fewer food cravings. She reported no adverse treatment-related effects.

Discussion

In my opinion, metabolic syndrome is frequently under-diagnosed in women. It is a combination of at least 3 or more of the following traits: high blood pressure (a value greater than 130/85), high levels of triglycerides (greater than or equal to 150 mg/dl) in the blood, a low level (less than or equal to 50 mg/dl) of HDL, a high fasting plasma glucose level (greater than or equal to 110), or abdominal obesity (a waist circumference of 35 inches or greater).[7]

Metabolic syndrome can contribute to the development of heart disease and diabetes. The syndrome may have a genetic basis, but its effects are intensified by factors that patients can control: a sedentary lifestyle; a diet high in fat, sugar, and calories; a high stress level; and alcohol or tobacco use.

It is important to remember that having a genetic predisposition to certain illnesses does not ensure that those diseases will develop. The human body has an amazing capability to overcome genetic disadvantages. When I was a medical student on rotation at the National Institutes of Health (NIH), I had the privilege of providing care for Pima Indian patients who participated in NIH-sponsored studies on diabetes.[8] Those studies showed that the Pima Indians who live in Arizona near the Gila River have an extremely high incidence of diabetes. About half of the Arizona Pimas are diabetic as adults, and about 80% who range in age from 55 to 65 years are diabetic. However, only about 1 in 15 adult Mexican Pimas, who descend from the same tribe and have the same genetic heritage as the Arizona Pimas, are diabetic.

Research has shown that although Pima Indians are genetically very susceptible to becoming diabetic, physical activity and a simple diet that is low in fat and high in fiber may prevent obesity, insulin resistance, and (ultimately) diabetes.[9] A research study of Mexican and Arizona Pimas showed that Mexican Pima men, whose diet was high in fiber and low in fat, spent an average of 29 hours per week performing moderate-to-heavy labor. Arizona Pima men devoted an average of 12 hours per week to that level of physical activity, but they ate a typical American diet (more than 35% fat, on average). The Mexican Pima men exhibited a lower rate of diabetes than did Arizona Pima men. The differences in diet and the level of physical activity level were thought to be responsible for the lower rate of diabetes in Mexican Pimas.[8]

In a recent article, experts on metabolic syndrome noted that many patients with that disorder are often treated with a collection of prescribed medications: Three or 4 drugs to lower the levels of cholesterol and triglycerides, 3 or 4 to control the level of blood glucose, and from 3 to 5 drugs to control blood pressure.[10] My approach to treating female patients with metabolic syndrome involves avoiding the high cost and potential adverse effects of multiple-drug therapy. Instead, I prefer to guide the patient in making corrective lifestyle changes and to write a prescription for only 1 medication: bioidentical progesterone. That hormone improves lipid values, lowers blood pressure, and improves the level of blood glucose (see Chapter 6). It is perhaps the most effective single agent for the treatment of metabolic syndrome in women.

References

1. Covington MB. Omega-3 fatty acids. *Am Fam Physician.* 2004;70(1):133-140.

2. Urizar NL, Liverman AB, Dodds DT, et al. A natural product that lowers cholesterol as an antagonist ligand for FXR. *Science.* 2002;296(5573):1703-1706. Epub: May 2, 2002.

3. Panda S, Kar A. Gugulu (Commiphora mukul) induces triiodothyronine production: possible involvement of lipid peroxidation. *Life Sci.* 1999;65(12):PL137-PL141.

4. Langsjoen PH, Langsjoen AM. Review of coenzyme Q10 in cardio-vascular disease with emphasis on heart failure and ischemia reperfusion. *Asia Pacific Heart J.* 1998;7(3):160-168.

5. Langsjoen PH, Langsjoen AM. Overview of the use of Co Q10 in cardiovascular disease. *Biofactors.* 1999;9(2-4):273-284.

6. Hu FB. The Mediterranean diet and mortality — olive oil and beyond. *N Engl J Med.* 2003;348(26):2595-2596.

7. Expert Panel on Detection, Evaluation, and Treatment of High Blood Cholesterol in Adults. Executive Summary of the Third Report of the National Cholesterol Education Program (NCEP) Expert Panel on Detection, Evaluation, and Treatment of High Blood Cholesterol in Adults (Adult Treatment Panel III). *JAMA.* 2001;16;285(19):2486-2497.

8. Esparza J, Fox C, Harper IT, et al. Daily energy expenditure in Mexican and USA Pima indians: low physical activity as a possible cause of obesity. *Int J Obes Relat Metab Disord.* 2000;24(1):55-59.

9. Williams DE, Knowler WC, Smith CJ, et al. The effect of Indian or Anglo dietary preference on the incidence of diabetes in Pima Indians. *Diabetes Care.* 2001;24(5):811-816.

10. Wise DE, Dewester J. Metabolic syndrome and associated cardio-vascular disease risk. *Am Acad Fam Physicians.* 2004;CME Bulletin 3(2):1-5.

Case 12. Painful Secrets

LL, a female patient in her late 40s, was admitted to the hospital for severe abdominal pain without associated nausea, vomiting, or bowel changes. She complained of sharp, intermittent, incapacitating waves of pain that occurred several times daily. When I examined LL, she writhed in pain when any degree of pressure was applied to her abdomen. Her husband was always present when she was examined. When the results of laboratory analyses and radiographic studies revealed no physical cause of the pain, I suspected that LL's abdominal discomfort might be psychogenic. After discussing her test results, I asked LL whether she had experienced recent stress or trauma. She glanced briefly at her husband and denied any such events. She then began complaining of abdominal pain and writhing in agony in her hospital bed. I ordered a few more studies and obtained a consultation from a surgeon. Although extensive evaluation revealed no physical cause of LL's discomfort, the surgeon was so impressed with the severity of her pain that he recommended exploratory abdominal surgery.

Later that morning, I asked LL again about stresses in her life, and she denied having any. My intuition suggested otherwise, and I resolved to return to her hospital room to talk with her alone late in the evening before the day of the scheduled exploratory surgery. When I arrived around 9:30 PM, I was slightly disappointed to see LL's husband sitting in her room. I greeted her and made some small talk. I then stated that I was concerned about whether the surgery scheduled for the next morning was the best decision. LL looked at her husband and asked, "Can I tell her?" The husband hesitated and then nodded. LL tearfully revealed that their only child, who was an adult living independently in another city, had recently visited them. During his visit, he had told them that he was gay and was openly living the gay lifestyle. LL said that this news was the worst thing she could ever imagine, and she refused to accept it. There was a stormy parting with her son. She was shocked and angered and felt that his homosexuality was a reflection of her failure as a mother.

In LL's cultural context, the gay lifestyle was considered to be a deviation, and she was convinced that her extended family and friends would reject her if they knew that she had a gay son. Many thoughts and feelings poured forth, and after an hour of sharing, she looked relaxed, her color had improved, and she asked whether I could cancel her surgery. I encouraged LL and her husband to talk about their son's coming out and reassured them that any true friend would not reject them because of his lifestyle. I also referred them for counseling both individually and as a couple. LL asked how it was possible that her emotional pain had caused such severe and genuine abdominal pain, and we discussed the power of the mind-body connection. Over the next few days and weeks, she continued to have a few brief episodes of pain, which gradually resolved. I recommended that she read *Women Who Run with the Wolves: Myths and Stories of the Wild Woman Archetype* (Pinkola Estés C. New York, NY: Ballantine Books; 1995) (especially the chapter on the "scar clan," which demonstrates that keeping secrets can make women ill) and *Anatomy of the Spirit: The Seven Stages of Power and Healing* (Myss C. New York, NY: Three Rivers Press; 1996), a discussion of mind-body connections in illness.

Case 13. Bedroom Problems

MM, a 51-year-old female patient, complained of daily headaches. She had been evaluated by many specialists and had undergone extensive testing and trials of different medications, but no cause of or treatment for her headache pain had been identified. She said that she had learned to adapt to her headaches by working at home on a flexible schedule. She denied changes in her diet, environment, exercise, and sleep quality. When I asked her specifically about her level of stress, she stated that her job was good, her adult children were independent and happy, and she had a stable marriage. She denied any stress over and above the usual daily challenges of work and household management.

At the time of her appointment, MM was being treated for chronic headaches with a combination of hydrocodone and acetaminophen (Vicodin), metaxalone (Skelaxin), and amitriptyline. She had undergone no prior surgeries, and her only illness had been chronic tension headaches. She had experienced 2 normal pregnancies with normal deliveries when she was in her 20s.

MM worked part-time in home-based employment. She lived with her husband and smoked 2 packs of cigarettes per day. Physical examination revealed tense muscle spasms in her neck and upper back.

Diagnosis
Chronic headaches

☞ Treatment
I agreed to prescribe medication for the headaches, but I emphasized the ultimate goal of nonreliance on daily medications. I also suggested that MM:

- Schedule a massage therapy session once weekly.

- Practice yoga 1 to 3 times weekly to reduce stress (see Chapter 3).

- Keep a diary of headache occurrence.

Follow Up
At her 6-week follow-up appointment, MM requested refills of her prescription medications. We again reviewed her lifestyle, work, relationships, and nutritional factors, and again no significant findings were noted. I asked her to complete a sandtray exercise (see Chapter 4) to guide both of us to sources of conflict in her life, because chronic headaches have been shown to occur as a result of psychologic stress.[1]

MM created a sandtray with a perfectly symmetrical circular arrangement of an angel figure, seashells, flowers, a flag, and a small lacquered box that was sealed shut.

She stated that the angel and flowers represented her mother, who had died when MM was a young girl. The seashells represented her attraction to the beach and the ocean. The flag symbolized her military service, and the box contained her physical and emotional pain. I felt that this exercise provided pertinent information about MM's early childhood trauma (the loss of her mother), but she did not think that there was a connection between her headache pain and the remote events symbolized in the sandtray exercise.

Secondary Follow Up

At her 6-week follow-up appointment, MM reported that her headache patterns had not changed. During that appointment, I asked again about her work, family, and home. She stated laughingly, "Well, everything is okay unless you believe in dreams." I said that I did believe that dreams contained important messages and asked MM whether she wanted to share one of her dream episodes. She then said that the dreams she had mentioned were not her own but those of her adult children. During the same week, both of her children reported having dreamed about their parents. One child had dreamed that MM and her husband were getting a divorce, and the other had dreamed that MM was having an affair. MM thought that both dreams were ridiculous; however, after further discussion she confided that her marriage was stressed because her husband was impotent. He insisted that she not reveal that aspect of their life. Before his impotence, MM and her husband had enjoyed a compatible sexual relationship. The onset of MM's daily headaches seemed to coincide with the loss of that aspect of her marriage. After further discussion, I felt that her husband might benefit from a medical evaluation and treatment, to which he eventually agreed.

The ability to openly discuss her husband's impotence brought relief to both MM and to her husband, whose therapy was successful. MM's headaches resolved as their marital stress diminished.

Reference

1. Stephenson K, Sparks T. Sand tray work in patient evaluation in a primary care environment. Paper presented at: First Biennial International Conference of Spirituality, Healing, and Health; April 10, 1999; Tucson, Ariz.

Case 14. Work That Makes You Sick

NN, a 53-year-old female patient, scheduled an appointment to ask questions about hormone replacement therapy (HRT). At the time of her appointment, she was being treated with synthetic estrogen, a therapy that was initiated 10 years earlier. She was experiencing mood swings, fatigue, intolerance to cold, aches and pains, and disturbed sleep. She suffered from allergic rhinitis and had undergone hysterectomy and oophorectomy 10 years earlier. Her medications included fluticasone (Flonase nasal), fexofenadine (Allegra), a calcium supplement, and a multivitamin. NN's mother had died of breast cancer that developed after menopause. Her father, who was in his 80s, enjoyed fair health, and her siblings were healthy.

At the time of her appointment, NN worked full-time as an executive secretary and lived with her husband, to whom she had been married for 30 years. She exercised 3 to 4 times weekly on a treadmill and denied alcohol and tobacco use.

NN admitted that she hated her work environment. I have observed that during midlife, women are more likely to experience tension when the values and practices in their workplace do not coincide with their core values. Because some women believe that they are less employable as they age, they endure unsatisfying work in an unpleasant environment and ultimately experience burnout.

NN's weight was in the low-normal range for her height. The results of her physical examination revealed mild fibrocystic change in her breasts, cold extremities, dry skin, and coarse, dry hair. Serum and saliva testing revealed the following results:

Serum testing (range)
> Thyroid hormones: Normal

Saliva testing (range)
> Estradiol: Normal
> Progesterone: Low
> Progesterone-estradiol ratio: Low
> Testosterone: Low
> Dehydroepiandrosterone sulfate (DHEAS): Low
> Cortisol: Morning - High
>> Noon - High
>> Evening - High
>> Bedtime - Low

Diagnosis
Estrogen dominance; deficiencies in progesterone, testosterone, and dehydroepiandrosterone (DHEA); adrenal dysfunction, workplace stress

☞ Treatment
Because NN preferred oral dosing, I prescribed the following treatment regimen:

- A combination of bioidentical hormones (80% estriol, 10% estradiol, and 10% estrone [Tri-Est] 2.5 mg plus bioidentical testosterone in oil capsule each morning) (see Chapter 6).

- Bioidentical progesterone 300 mg (1 tablet at bedtime) (see Chapter 6).

- Increased consumption of broccoli, cauliflower, cabbage, citrus, and tomatoes (foods that may protect against cancer).

- Continuing use of a calcium supplement and a multivitamin.

- Practicing yoga 3 times weekly in addition to her current treadmill program (see Chapter 3).

- Keeping a diary of symptoms.

- Scheduling a Bio-Touch session once weekly (see Chapter 7).

- Planning lunch breaks and midday breaks to interrupt a stressful work environment and create serenity during the work day.

- Completing a handwork project (see Chapter 5).

- Creating a "self-awareness" shirt by using red and black fabric markers to write personal affirmations that evoke feelings of hope, self-worth, and encouragement on the *inside* of a white tuxedo shirt, which can be purchased at many craft shops. Red, black, and white are traditional colors that represent the maiden (white), the woman (red), and the wise woman (black), which embody the progressive stages of a woman's life. When a woman wearing a self-awareness shirt stands before a mirror, she can read the quotations written on the inside of the garment. At that moment, she literally stands behind the words she has selected to remind her of her purpose, goals, and dreams. For my self-awareness shirt, I used quotations found in 2 books by Sarah Ban Breathnach: *Simple Abundance: A Daybook of Comfort and Joy* (New York, NY: Warner Books; 1995) and *Romancing the Ordinary: A*

Year of Simple Splendor (New York, NY: Simple Abundance Press/Scribner; 2002).

- Journaling; writing down work-related conflicts that NN could not discuss because of job-security issues. The journals could be periodically shredded or burned in NN's fireplace while she relaxed with a glass of wine or a cup of cocoa.

☞ **Cinematherapy**
- *Working Girl*

- *9 to 5*

☞ **Suggested reading**
Hoff B. *The Tao of Pooh*. New York, NY: Penguin Books; 1983.

Lee JR, Zava D, Hopkins H. *What Your Doctor May Not Tell You About Breast Cancer: How Hormone Balance Can Save Your Life*. New York, NY: Warner Books, Inc; 2002.

Wilson JL. *Adrenal Fatigue: The 21st Century Stress Syndrome*. Petaluma, Calif: Smart Publications; 2001. Web site: www.adrenalfatigue.org.

Williamson M. *A Woman's Worth*. New York, NY: Random House, 1993.

Follow up
At her 12-week follow-up appointment, NN reported improved sleep and mood and fewer aches and pains. She continued to experience fatigue, cold intolerance, and decreased libido. Her hair and skin remained dry. Results of repeat saliva testing revealed that all abnormal hormone values were within the normal range with the exception of cortisol, the level of which remained high in the morning, at noon, and in the evening.

Secondary Diagnosis
Functional thyroid deficiency (see Chapter 6)

☞ *Treatment Modification*
- Thyroid tablets, USP (Armour thyroid) 15 mg (1 tablet once daily in the morning).

- Adherence to the original treatment regimen described above and the use of stress-reduction techniques in the workplace

Secondary Follow Up
At her 8-week follow-up appointment, NN stated that her symptoms were much improved. She had noticed a reduction in cold intolerance, more moisture in her hair and skin, fewer aches and pains, and improved libido.

Discussion
Stress in the workplace can adversely affect the health of women employees, but many working women in midlife are reluctant to speak up or resign because their job is a necessity. Finding creative and healthful ways of coping with workplace stress can help many women to get through the work week. Participating in a weekly yoga class can benefit emotional and physical health and reduce stress (see Chapter 3). Bio-Touch therapy (see Chapter 7), which requires no special equipment or supplies, can be performed in the workplace to provide needed relief from stress. After I had trained Bio-Touch practitioners at our health center, I noticed that many of our female employees had begun to meet to exchange Bio-Touch on their breaks or would call a schedule a session to obtain relief from headache, neck pain, or menstrual cramps. Women connecting to each other in a healthful way can induce positive changes even in a workplace where high stress is the norm.

Case 15. The Domineering Mother
OO, a 54-year-old female patient, requested treatment with bioidentical hormone replacement therapy (BHRT).

Ten years earlier, she had been diagnosed as having rheumatoid arthritis. She had undergone hysterectomy and the removal of both ovaries 20 years earlier and had been treated since that time with injections of estradiol cypionate (Depo-Estradiol) every 3 weeks to relieve menopausal symptoms. She stated that she had long experienced relief from those symptoms for 4 weeks after each hormone injection. About 18 months earlier, however, she had begun to suffer from mood swings, headaches, weight gain, sugar cravings, frequent urinary tract infections, and hot flashes early in the third week after each injection.

At the time of her office visit, OO was being treated with methotrexate, levothyroxine sodium (Levoxyl), esomeprazole magnesium (Nexium), calcium, vitamins E and C, and a multivitamin with B complex in addition to the injections of the Depo-Estradiol that relieved her menopausal symptoms. She had been diagnosed as having hypothyroidism and gastroesophageal reflux. She had never been pregnant and had been evaluated and treated for infertility with various fertility drugs when she was in her 20s. OO had undergone several orthopedic surgeries to correct the effects of severe rheumatoid arthritis. Her mother, who was in her 70s, was healthy, as were OO's siblings.

OO was divorced. Because of her severe rheumatoid arthritis, she was unable to maintain employment or to be independent. She had moved into an apartment on her mother's property but found that arrangement to be highly stressful because her mother was very intrusive. She would continually violate OO's privacy by reading her mail, rearranging her furniture, and openly criticizing many aspects of OO's life (her clothing, spending habits, choice of friends, housekeeping ability, cooking skills, and church attendance). OO stated that her mother criticized and belittled her in most of their inter-actions, and OO responded deferentially. She had never become an adult child in her relationship with her mother.

OO did not exercise, and she was obese. Her hands and feet had been deformed by rheumatoid arthritis. She smoked about half a pack of cigarettes per day and stated that her diet was poor because she avoided eating meals with her mother and did not want to cook just for herself. She enjoyed the companionship of her dog, however.

During physical examination, fibrocystic changes in both breasts and thinning of vaginal and vulvar tissue were detected. Serum and saliva testing revealed the following results:

Serum testing (range)
> Thyroid hormones: Normal

Saliva testing (range)
> Estradiol: High
> Progesterone: Low
> Progesterone-estradiol ratio: Low
> Testosterone: Low
> Dehydroepiandrosterone sulfate (DHEAS): Normal
> Cortisol: Morning - High
> > Noon - Normal
> > Evening - Normal
> > Bedtime - Normal

Diagnosis

Estrogen dominance, progesterone and testosterone deficiency, rheumatoid arthritis, atrophic vaginitis, hypothyroidism, gastroesophageal reflux, obesity, adrenal dysfunction

☞ Treatment

- A combination of bioidentical hormones (80% estriol and 20% estradiol [Bi-Est] 1.25 mg plus bioidentical testosterone 5 mg in oil) (1 capsule daily) (see Chapter 6).

- Reducing the frequency of and then terminating treatment with Depo-Estradiol injections over a 2-month period.

- Bioidentical progesterone 400 mg (1 extended-release tablet at bedtime) (see Chapter 6).

- Bioidentical estriol vaginal suppositories 1 mg (1 suppository at bedtime for 3 days, then twice weekly at bedtime) (see Chapter 6).

- Gradually eliminating fast-food consumption and more frequently preparing meals at home or with friends.

- Practicing "bedtop" yoga (see Chapter 3).

- Scheduling a Bio-Touch session once weekly (see Chapter 7).

- Keeping a diary of symptoms.

- Volunteering in the community 4 hours weekly.

☞ Cinematherapy
- *Like Water for Chocolate*

- *Drop Dead Fred*

☞ Suggested reading
Love P, Robinson J. *The Emotional Incest Syndrome: What To Do When a Parent's Love Rules Your Life.* New York, NY: Bantam Books; 1990.

Bolen JS. *Ring of Power: The Abandoned Child, The Authoritarian Father, and the Disempowered Feminine: A Jungian Understanding of Wagner's Ring Cycle*. San Francisco, Calif: HarperSanFrancisco; 1992.

Engel B. *The Emotionally Abused Woman: Overcoming Destructive Patterns and Reclaiming Yourself*. New York, NY: Ballantine Books; 1992.

Follow Up

At her 12-week follow-up appointment, OO reported fewer headaches and hot flashes. Her craving for sugar had diminished. Twenty-four weeks after the initiation of the recommended therapies, she said, "I feel better than I have felt in years." She had lost 15 pounds and felt well enough to begin working part-time. She had begun to set limits and establish emotional boundaries with her mother and was making long-term plans to live independently.

Discussion

In clinical practice, I have noted a strong association between a low testosterone level and connective tissue diseases in women. The identification and treatment of testosterone deficiency in women with a connective tissue disease can make a significant difference in relieving or improving pain, fatigue, sleep disturbances, and stamina. I also felt that OO's health problems were intensified by her toxic relationship with her mother.

Case 16. Fibroids, Cysts, and Hormones

PP, a 55-year-old female patient, sought consultation about the use of hormone replacement therapy (HRT). She had been treated with conjugated equine estrogens and medroxyprogesterone acetate (Prempro) for 5 years but stopped therapy with that drug abruptly after the National Heart, Lung, and Blood Institute Women's Health Initiative (WHI) trials were terminated early. She was treating her menopausal symptoms with over-the-counter herbal formulas (black cohosh, Siberian ginseng, wild yam extract, dong quai, licorice root) but continued to experience hot flashes, mood swings, heavy menstrual periods, and bloating. Her obstetrician-gynecologist had recommended that PP undergo hysterectomy, but she was strongly opposed to having surgery and wanted a trial of nonsurgical options. Her hormone levels had never been evaluated.

For 3 years, PP had had high blood pressure, which was treated with triamterene plus hydrochlorothiazide (Maxzide). Episodes of allergic rhinitis were controlled with cetirizine hydrochloride (Zyrtec) as needed. In her 20s, she had experienced 2 normal pregnancies with normal deliveries and had then undergone tubal ligation. She had gained 30 pounds over the last 5 years.

PP's mother, who had experienced menopause at 59 years of age, died of breast cancer. Her maternal aunt and maternal cousin also suffered from breast cancer. Her father died of complications from Alzheimer's disease.

At the time of her appointment, PP was divorced and lived alone. She worked 16 hours daily in her small business. She drank 1 to 2 glasses of wine weekly and did not smoke. She did not exercise and stated that she ate a high-fat diet.

During physical examination, abdominal obesity, an enlarged uterus, and fibrocystic changes in both breasts were detected. PP's blood pressure was within the normal range. A complete blood count showed moderately severe anemia. Serum and saliva testing and other medical evaluations revealed the following results:

Serum testing (range)
> Thyroid hormones: Normal
> Serum lipid profile: Normal

Saliva testing (range)
> Estradiol: High
> Progesterone: Low
> Progesterone-estradiol: Low
> Testosterone: Normal
> Dehydroepiandrosterone sulfate (DHEAS): Normal
> Cortisol: Morning - Normal
> Evening - Normal

Other medical evaluations
Endometrial biopsy: No precancerous or cancerous changes in the uterine lining
Pelvic ultrasonography: Enlarged uterus with a small fibroid tumor, small cysts on both ovaries

Diagnosis
Estrogen dominance, progesterone deficiency, heavy menstrual periods, a small uterine fibroid tumor, benign ovarian cysts, anemia, obesity, high blood pressure

☞ Treatment
Because PP requested oral dosing, I prescribed the following treatment regimen:

- Bioidentical progesterone extended-release tablets 400 mg (1 tablet twice daily) (see Chapter 6).

- Iron supplement daily.

- Following the Mediterranean diet.

- Practicing yoga 1 to 3 times weekly (see Chapter 3).

- Increasing physical activity during the workday.

- Keeping a diary of symptoms.

- Completing a handwork project (see Chapter 5).

☞ Suggested reading

Lee JR, Zava D, Hopkins H. *What Your Doctor May Not Tell You About Breast Cancer: How Hormone Balance Can Save Your Life.* New York, NY: Warner Books, Inc; 2002.

Northrup C. *Women's Bodies, Women's Wisdom: Creating Physical and Emotional Health and Healing.* New York, NY: Bantam Books; 1994.

Spangle L. *Life Is Hard, Food Is Easy: The 5-Step Plan To Overcome Emotional Eating and Lose Weight on Any Diet.* Washington, DC: LifeLine Press; 2003.

☞ Internet resources

www.oldwayspt.org — Information about the Mediterranean diet.

www.tops.org — TOPS (Take Off Pounds Sensibly) support group.

Follow Up

At her 8-week follow-up visit, PP reported no adverse effects from treatment with progesterone, and she had made changes in her lifestyle and diet. She was experiencing heavy menstrual periods less frequently. We discussed increasing her dosage of oral progesterone, but PP was concerned about the cost of that medication.

☞ Treatment Modification

- Topical bioidentical progesterone cream 120 mg/mL (0.3 mL to be applied to a thin-skinned area such as the inner thigh or inner arm twice daily).

Secondary Follow Up

At her 14-week follow-up appointment, PP reported that her menstrual periods had become normal. Laboratory analysis showed that her anemia had partially resolved. She had lost 10 pounds.

Tertiary Follow Up

At her 26-week follow-up appointment, PP stated that she had noted an improvement in all symptoms. Her anemia had resolved, and she had lost an additional 20 pounds.

Discussion

Hormone imbalances can contribute to changes in menstrual patterns and flow. Obesity and a high-fat diet can worsen such imbalances. PP was able to meet her goal of avoiding surgical treatment for heavy menstrual bleeding by taking bioidentical progesterone, implementing nutritional changes, and losing weight.

Case 17. Putting on the Red Hat

QQ, a 55-year-old woman, presented with a request for bioidentical hormone replacement therapy (BHRT). After having undergone hysterectomy and the removal of both ovaries 20 years earlier, she had been treated with multiple hormone-containing preparations, including esterified estrogens and methyltestosterone (Estratest), conjugated equine estrogens (Premarin), and transdermal estradiol (Climara), as well as various herbal remedies to relieve severe menopausal symptoms. QQ stated that when she was taking those hormone replacements, she "never felt right" and continued to experience night sweats so severe that her nightclothes and pillowcase were drenched with perspiration. The night sweats interrupted her sleep, and when she awoke, her thoughts would race. She would ruminate about what she should have done, had to do, was unable to do, etc. She slept only a few hours per night.

QQ had experienced midbody weight gain. She complained of fatigue, intolerance to cold, dry hair and skin, an increased frequency of aches and pains, decreased libido, and vaginal dryness.

At the time of her appointment, QQ was treating pain from arthritis with valdecoxib (Bextra) as needed. She also took a daily multivitamin and additional vitamins C and E. Her only prior illness was postpregnancy thyroiditis for which she was treated with ablation. She had undergone 3 normal pregnancies with normal deliveries when she was in her 20s. Her only prior surgery was hysterectomy and the removal of both ovaries for the treatment of uterine fibroid tumors. QQ's parents were in their 80s. Her father suffered from heart disease, as did her brother. Her mother had osteoporosis.

When she became my patient, QQ was living with her husband and owned a small business. She drank 2 to 3 glasses of wine per week and did not smoke. She exercised sporadically by following a walking program. She often prepared homecooked meals that included lean meats, fresh fruits, and vegetables. QQ provided for the daily needs and medical requirements of her parents, who lived nearby. She mentioned having frequent conflicts with her adult daughters.

Physical examination revealed that QQ's weight was normal for her height and that her thyroid was enlarged. Changes in her large joints suggested osteoarthritis, and thinning of vulvar and vaginal tissues was noted. Serum and saliva testing revealed the following results:

Serum testing (range)
> Thyroid-stimulating hormone (TSH): High normal
> Free levothyroxine (T_4): Low normal
> Cholesterol: Normal

Saliva testing (range)
> Estradiol: Low
> Progesterone: Low
> Progesterone-estradiol ratio: Low
> Testosterone: Low
> Dehydroepiandrosterone sulfate (DHEAS): Normal

Cortisol: Morning - High
       Noon: Low
       Evening: Normal
       Bedtime: High

Diagnosis

Deficiency of estrogen, progesterone, and testosterone; adrenal dysfunction; subclinical hypothyroidism; osteoarthritis; atrophic vaginitis

☞ Treatment

Because QQ requested oral dosing, I prescribed the following regimen:

- A combination of the following bioidentical hormones in an extended-release tablet: 80% estriol and 20% estradiol (Bi-Est) 2.5 mg, testosterone 4 mg, and progesterone 300 mg (1 tablet once daily or a half tablet in the morning and a half tablet in the evening) (see Chapter 6).

- Bioidentical estriol vaginal suppositories 1 mg (1 suppository at bedtime for 3 days, then 1 suppository twice weekly) (see Chapter 6).

- Traumeel Ointment (Heel Biotherapeutics, Heel Canada Inc, Montreal, Quebec), a homeopathic preparation for painful joints. Traumeel can be ordered by a pharmacist.

- Thyroid tablets, USP (Armour thyroid) 15 mg (1 tablet each morning for 3 weeks, then 2 tablets [a total of 30 mg] each morning as a maintenance dosage) (see Chapter 6).

- A daily calcium supplement containing vitamin D and magnesium.

- Practicing yoga 1 to 3 times weekly (see Chapter 3).

- Scheduling a Bio-Touch session once weekly (see Chapter 7).

- Keeping a diary of symptoms.

- Completing a handwork project (see Chapter 5).

✿ Suggested reading

Bassoff E. *Mothers and Daughters: Loving and Letting Go.* New York, NY: New American Library; 1988.

Bolen JS. *Crossing to Avalon: A Woman's Midlife Pilgrimage.* San Francisco, Calif: HarperSanFrancisco; 1994.

Bolen JS. *Goddesses in Everywoman: A New Psychology of Women.* New York, NY: Harper & Row; 1984.

Lee JR, Zava D, Hopkins H. *What Your Doctor May Not Tell You About Breast Cancer: How Hormone Balance Can Save Your Life.* New York, NY: Warner Books, Inc; 2002.

Follow Up

At her 8-week follow-up appointment, QQ reported no treatment-related adverse effects. She stated that she felt better when she divided the BHRT into twice-daily doses, half in the morning and half in the evening. She felt better overall, and the quality of her sleep had improved. Her mood was more calm, and she had noticed an improvement in sexual arousal and orgasm. She had recently been emotionally stressed by the critical illness and prolonged hospitalization of her father in addition to increased business demands, so she had not been exercising.

At her 16-week follow-up appointment, salivary testing revealed that all hormone levels were within the normal range, as were the levels of thyroid hormones. QQ had begun to exercise and reported that all symptoms had improved.

Discussion

For some women, the transition to menopause is a time of intense physical and psychologic adjustment in a society that values youth and beauty. Understanding the changes that occur during menopause and connecting with other menopausal women are helpful for those individuals. The Red Hat Society, a social group for women older than 50 years, can be found in most US cities.

Women like QQ who have severe menopausal symptoms may not feel well if they are treated with standardized doses of synthetic hormones. However, their menopausal symptoms may require medical treatment if herbal therapies, changes in lifestyle, and dietary modifications do not produce relief. BHRT provides the patient with hormones that more closely mimic those produced by the human body. I have observed that women treated with BHRT experience the benefits of hormone supplementation but fewer adverse effects.

Case 18. Heart Break

RR, a woman in her mid-50s, had been my patient for several years. Her high blood pressure was controlled with medication. She was postmenopausal and had elected not to take hormone replacement. RR smoked 1 pack of cigarettes daily. She worked as a nurse. She stated that her marriage was very unhappy because her husband was unfaithful, but she had chosen to remain married for the sake of her children and to preserve the family unit. RR admitted to being very lonely and said that she often went to movies or to dinner alone. She was too ashamed of her husband's infidelity to confide in a friend.

I saw RR a few times each year for wellness evaluations and to treat minor illnesses. One day, she called my office to ask for an appointment. She stated that all morning while she had been at work, she had been feeling a "ping" in her chest. Because my receptionist wasn't sure what RR was describing, she wisely transferred the call to my nurse. The nurse was concerned because RR seldom called the office and because she was at risk for cardiovascular disease. The nurse urged her to come to the office immediately for an evaluation, but like many dedicated women, RR did not want to leave her job at midday. She stated that she did not want to "dump her workload on someone else" and felt that she could wait until the end of her shift to come to the office for examination. In the late afternoon she did so, and the results of her electrocardiogram were abnormal.

Diagnosis
Coronary artery disease

☞ Treatment
I admitted RR to the hospital and consulted a cardiologist about her condition. Further examination revealed extensive heart blockages that required cardiac bypass surgery, and RR underwent immediate cardiac catheterization.

Follow Up
By the time of her 12-week follow-up appointment, RR had completed a cardiac rehabilitation program and was able to return to work. She agreed to begin counseling and, as part of that intervention, she began to engage in hobbies and social interactions with friends and groups who shared her interests

Discussion
This case illustrates what I refer to as "the 7 Ds of heart disease in women":

Difficulty in diagnosis. Women do not tend to exhibit the classic symptoms of heart disease that are defined in men. RR, for example, never complained of chest pain or pressure. She instead accurately described an unusual sensation that caused her concern. A recent study showed that the 2 symptoms most strongly correlated with heart attacks in women are disturbed sleep and fatigue, both of which occurred during the month before the event.[1-5] Such vague nonspecific complaints are often dismissed by the patient as being due to stress or by the physician as being insignificant.

Delay in treatment. In the United States, the mortality rate from heart attack is higher in women than men for several reasons. Like RR, many women tend to delay seeking medical care. Others hope that their symptoms will subside, or they may fear that by expressing health-related concerns they will become a burden to friends or family members. In some women who seek medical care, the diagnosis of cardiovascular disease and appropriate treatment may be delayed because women have communication styles, symptoms of cardiac disease, and physiologic function that are different from those in men, who are the subjects of most cardiovascular disease research.[2-4]

Disparity. As stated above, more women than men in the United States die of cardiovascular disease each year, and in 2000 nearly twice as many US women died from cardiovascular disease than from all cancers combined.[6,7] When asked about their most serious health concern, women are more likely to state a fear of cancer rather than cardiovascular disease.[5]

Differences in cardiac physiology. Only in the last decade, when the mandated inclusion of women in research studies and drug trials was implemented, have researchers begun to illuminate the gender differences in the anatomy and physiology of the heart.

Depression and despair. Persistent unrelieved psychologic stress in women has been linked to an increased risk of heart disease. RR had experienced significant stress in her marriage and at work.

Disability. After having undergone cardiac bypass surgery, women are less likely than men to return to their previous employment status or level of function.[8] There are several explanations for that difference. Women patients tend to participate less often in cardiac rehabilitation programs than do men, or they are reluctant to engage in small-group rehabilitation in which most of the other patients are men. Obtaining transportation is a problem for some women, and still others feel that they must use their financial resources for the needs of other family members.

Death. Women are more likely than men to die of heart disease.[4,6,7] After coronary bypass surgery, women are also more likely than men to die. In women who have undergone that procedure, research shows that those 59 years or younger have the greatest risk of death.[9]

References

1. Rathore SS, Chen J, Wang Y, Radford MJ, Vaccarino V, Krumholz HM. Sex differences in cardiac catheterization: the role of physician gender. *JAMA.* 2001;286(22):2849-2856.

2. Gibler WB, Armstrong PW, Ohman EM, et al. Global Use of Strategies to Open Occluded Coronary Arteries (GUSTO) Investigators. Persistence of delays in presentation and treatment for patients with acute myocardial infarction: the GUSTO-I and GUSTO-III experience. *Ann Emerg Med.* 2002;39(2):123-130.

3. Arnold AL, Milner KA, Vaccarino V. Sex and race differences in electrocardiogram use (the National Hospital Ambulatory Medical Care Survey). *Am J Cardiol.* 2001;88(9):1037-1040.

4. Vakili BA, Kaplan RC, Brown DL. Sex-based differences in early mortality of patients undergoing primary angioplasty for first acute myocardial infarction. *Circulation.* 2001;104(25):3034-3038.

5. Marcuccio E, Loving N, Bennett SK, Hayes SN. A survey of attitudes and experiences of women with heart disease. *Womens*

Health Issues. 2003;13(1):23-31.

6. American Heart Association Women. Heart disease and stroke statistics — 2003. Available at: www.americanheart.org. Accessed July 2, 2004.

7. American Heart Association. Women and cardiovascular disease biostatistical fact sheet. Available at: www.americanheart.org. Accessed July 2, 2004.

8. Vaccarino V, Lin ZQ, Kasl SV, et al. Gender differences in recovery after coronary artery bypass surgery. *J Am Coll Cardiol.* 2003;41(2):307-314.

9. Vaccarino V, Abramson JL, Veledar E, Weintraub WS. Sex differences in hospital mortality after coronary artery bypass surgery: evidence for a higher mortality in younger women. *Circulation.* 2002;105(10):1176-1181.

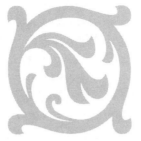

Appendix C:
Case Reports — Midlife and Beyond

Athena chose the owl as her favorite bird. She was often depicted with the little owl Athene noctua, her pet and companion, at her side. According to Greek mythology, the owl possessed a magical inner light that was the source of its extraordinary night vision. Owls were featured on the Greek coins used in trade. When engraved on jewelry, they were thought to protect the wearer and to ensure victory in battle. The owl has remained a symbol of mystery and power in many cultures. In Native American legends, it is referred to as "the watcher of the dark." Often portrayed as a guardian, the owl is also associated with death and is thought of as a guide from the earthly realm to the spiritual realm. Women at midlife and beyond have the capacity to serve others as a guide and guardian. Those who nurture their inner light and cultivate the awareness of their role as guardian and guide become a source of strength and support for others.

This chapter is dedicated to Alice L. Cooke, PhD, who was my employer and mentor when I attended The University of Texas. She personified the Athenian ideal in all aspects of her life and work.

Dr. Cooke was the first female English professor at The University of Texas, from which she retired after a lengthy and successful career. I first met Dr. Cooke when she was in her early 90s. She required constant assistance with personal care because of health problems, and she employed several women (of which I was one) to fulfill that role. She enjoyed a long and happy marriage but had been widowed for several years when I met her. She had no children.

The work of Walt Whitman was the subject of Dr. Cooke's thesis, and she often quoted from Leaves of Grass. *Although she suffered from physical limitations caused by a stroke, heart disease, and a hip fracture, her spirit and intellect were very active. Even as she lived with the awareness of being close to death, she enjoyed daily life. She took pleasure in listening to music. She was an avid sports fan and especially enjoyed baseball, golf, and football. She delighted in having her hair styled and her nails manicured. Dr. Cooke was also a fierce player in weekly bridge games that, because she could not travel, were held in her home in Hyde Park. Before each game, card tables were placed in her formal dining room. Refreshments were served on fine china, and glasses of sherry were always offered to her guests.*

Dr. Cooke was known for her ready wit and her great sense of humor. She enjoyed telling stories about her childhood; the early development of Austin, Texas; and university life. She was a guardian and advisor to the women whom she employed and to her friends and extended family. Exceptionally perceptive in assessing situations and individuals, she eloquently dispensed words of wisdom as well as warning. A trusted friend and teacher, she was always glad to share her experience and her time, which endeared her to students. She was an imposing employer, but I liked and admired her tremendously, and our friendship grew during the 3 years that I worked for her. Dr. Alice

Cooke was an excellent role model who shaped for the better the life, career, and future of many young women.

Rather than detailing the many treatments often required to preserve health in later life, the case reports in this chapter focus on the wisdom, resilience, and spirituality of older women. Through the choices they made, many of the women profiled here transformed their life for the better and proved indeed that it is never too late. Like Dr. Cooke, women beyond midlife have the power to transform the lives of others through their role as guide and guardian.

Case 1. The "Premrose" Path

AA, a 61-year-old female patient, sought a second opinion about the safety of hormone replacement therapy (HRT). She had been treated with conjugated equine estrogens plus medroxyprogesterone acetate (Prempro) for a few years before she underwent hysterectomy and the removal of both ovaries. After that surgery, she was treated with conjugated equine estrogens (Premarin) for 10 years. She said that she had been scolded by her physician for recently stopping treatment with Premarin. AA reported that during the prior decade, her health had progressively worsened. Her current symptoms included weight gain in the waist, hips, and thighs; thinning scalp hair; migraines; joint and muscle pain; fibrocystic breasts; fatigue; food cravings; and irritable mood.

At the time of her appointment, AA was being treated with atorvastatin calcium (Lipitor) to lower her levels of cholesterol and triglycerides, which had been elevated for 8 years; enalapril maleate (Vasotec) to control high blood pressure diagnosed 5 years earlier; celecoxib (Celebrex) to relieve joint pain; sertraline (Zoloft) (AA was not certain why this drug had been prescribed); zolpidem tartrate (Ambien) to relieve insomnia; sumatriptan (Imitrex) to treat migraines; and pantoprazole (Protonix) to control gastroesophageal reflux. She also took a calcium supplement and a multivitamin daily.

AA had undergone multiple biopsies of breast lesions, which proved to be benign. She said that she dreaded undergoing mammograms, the results of which were always abnormal. She had experienced 2 normal pregnancies with normal deliveries. Her mother, who suffered from osteoporosis, died in a motor vehicle accident when she was in her 70s. Her father had suffered from colon cancer and had had a stroke, but her siblings were healthy. AA lived with her husband, who had recently retired. She had attended college and did not work outside the home. She stated that she occasionally drank wine, did not smoke, and followed a low-fat diet. She was, however, clinically obese. She exercised by participating in a walking program.

Physical examination revealed marked thinning of scalp hair, fibrocystic changes in both breasts, and osteoarthritis of the hands and knees. Serum and saliva testing revealed the following results:

Serum testing (range)
>   Thyroid hormones: Normal
>   Glucose: Slightly elevated
>   Triglycerides: High
>   Total cholesterol: High

Saliva testing (range)
>   Estradiol: Normal
>   Progesterone: Normal
>   Progesterone-estrogen ratio: Low
>   Testosterone: Normal
>   Dehydroepiandrosterone sulfate (DHEAS): Normal
>   Cortisol: Morning - High
>   Bedtime - High

Diagnosis

Estrogen dominance, progesterone deficiency, adrenal dysfunction, obesity, metabolic syndrome, high blood pressure, high levels of total cholesterol and triglycerides, insomnia, migraines, gastroesophageal reflux

☞ Treatment

- Topical bioidentical progesterone cream 20 mg/mL (1 mL to be applied to a thin-skinned area such as the inner arm or inner thigh at bedtime) (see Chapter 6).

- Termination of treatment with Lipitor and Ambien, because progesterone can lower the levels of triglycerides and can improve sleep.

- Fish oil (3 g daily in capsule form).[1]

- Guggul extract to improve the levels of triglycerides and cholesterol and enhance thyroid function.[2,3]

- Coenzyme Q_{10} for cardiovascular protection.[4,5]

- Traumeel Ointment (Heel Biotherapeutics, Heel Canada Inc, Montreal, Quebec), a homeopathic preparation, to treat painful joints. Traumeel can be ordered by a pharmacist.

- Changing the beverage of choice to water.

- Adhering to the Mediterranean diet and noting the glycemic index of foods consumed.

- Practicing yoga and continuing the walking program (see Chapter 3).

- Scheduling a Bio-Touch session once weekly (see Chapter 7).

- Keeping a diary of symptoms and foods consumed.

- Completing a handwork project (see Chapter 5).

☞ Cinematherapy
- *About Schmidt*

- *Cocoon*

☞ Suggested reading
Lee JR, Zava D, Hopkins H. *What Your Doctor May Not Tell You About Breast Cancer: How Hormone Balance Can Save Your Life.* New York, NY: Warner Books, Inc; 2002

Wilson JL. *Adrenal Fatigue: The 21st Century Stress Syndrome.* Petaluma, Calif: Smart Publications; 2001. Web site: www.adrenalfatigue.org

☞ Internet resources
www.salivatest.com — A link to ZRT Laboratory, which provides saliva testing

www.adrenalfatigue.org — A link to a Web site offering information about adrenal fatigue

www.oldwayspt.org/pyramids — A link to a Web site offering information about the Mediterranean diet

Follow Up
Four weeks later, AA reported a dramatic improvement in her symptoms. She was experiencing less breast tenderness and had noted the growth of new scalp hair. Her sleep and mood had improved. She had lost 5 pounds. I recommended that AA taper off treatment with Zoloft because she did not know why the drug had been prescribed, and I felt that it was contributing to her decreased libido.

Secondary Follow Up
At her follow-up appointment 4 months after having initiated the recommended changes, AA was barely rec-

ognizable. She had a new hairstyle and was wearing tailored clothing that accentuated her slimmer figure. She reported a continuing improvement in her symptoms. Her hair and skin had more luster. She had noted increased stamina and muscle contouring and improved sleep and mood. She experienced renewed vitality and a sense of well-being. She had lost 25 pounds and was continuing to exercise regularly by walking and practicing yoga. She no longer experienced headaches. Her joint pain was greatly diminished, and she had stopped taking Celebrex. As a result of her change in diet and her weight loss, she no longer suffered from gastroesophageal reflux and had stopped treatment with Protonix. However, she had experienced some lightheadedness and stated that her blood pressure was often low when she monitored it at home. Serum and saliva testing revealed the following values:

Serum testing (range)
> Triglycerides: Normal
> Total cholesterol: Normal
> Glucose: Normal

Saliva testing (range)
> Estradiol: Normal
> Progesterone: Normal
> Estradiol-progesterone ratio: Normal
> Testosterone: Normal
> Dehydroepiandrosterone sulfate (DHEAS): Normal
> Cortisol: Morning - Improved
> Bedtime - Normal

☞ **Treatment Modification**
Stop treatment with Vasotec (which controls high blood pressure) because AA's high blood pressure had resolved.

Discussion

In my opinion, AA exhibited premenopausal estrogen dominance that was worsened by treatment with Prempro and Premarin. In addition, her downward health spiral reflected the known effects of estrogen dominance (elevated levels of triglycerides, migraines, and weight gain that contributed to osteoarthritis and gastroesophageal reflux). AA was highly motivated to improve her health and wanted to decrease the number of prescription medications that she was taking, several of which are the most often prescribed drugs in the United States (see Chapter 6). By following the "test-and-treat" approach and changing her diet and lifestyle over 6 months, she successfully discontinued the use of all prescribed medications except bioidentical progesterone and was enjoying a better quality of health and life.

References

1. Covington MB. Omega-3 Fatty Acids. *Am Fam Physician.* 2004;70(1):133-140.

2. Urizar NL, Liverman AB, Dodds DT, et al. A natural product that lowers cholesterol as an antagonist ligand for the FXR. *Science.* 2002;296(5573):1703-1706.

3. Panda S, Kar A. Gugulu (Commiphora mukul) induces triiodothyronine production: possible involvement of lipid peroxidation. *Life Sci.* 1999;65(12):PL137-PL141.

4. Langsjoen PH, Langsjoen AM. Coenzyme Q10 in cardiovascular disease with emphasis on heart failure and ischemia reperfusion. *Asia Pacific Heart J.* 1998;7(3):160-168.

5. Langsjoen PH, Langsjoen AM. Overview of the use of CoQ10 in cardiovascular disease. *Biofactors.* 1999;9(2-4):273-284.

Case 2. Hormones and Heart Disease

BB, a 62-year-old woman, complained of the following symptoms: hot flashes that occurred during the day and at night; night sweats; fatigue; weight gain in the abdomen, hips, and thighs; a craving for sugar; dry skin and hair; and a feeling of decreased intellectual sharpness.

Those symptoms, which were severe, interfered with her work and diminished her quality of life. She often had to change clothes at work because hot flashes left her drenched with perspiration. She was told by her former physician that she could not receive hormone therapy because she had heart disease.

At the time of her office visit, BB was receiving treatment with triamterene and hydrochlorothiazide (Maxzide), atorvastatin (Lipitor), aspirin, coenzyme Q_{10}, a daily multivitamin, and a daily calcium supplement. Six months earlier, she had suffered a heart attack that was treated by stent placement to prevent blockage of her coronary artery. After having undergone that procedure, she stopped treatment with conjugated estrogens (Premarin) as her physician had advised. BB had undergone hysterectomy and the removal of both ovaries when she was in her 40s. She had experienced 3 normal pregnancies and normal deliveries when she was in her 20s. Her mother had died of a stroke and her father, of a heart attack. Her brother had high blood pressure and diabetes.

BB lived with her spouse and owned her own business. She did not drink alcohol or smoke, and she followed a low-fat diet. She was, however, obese. Her score on the Beck Depression Inventory Depression Scale was in the normal range. Saliva testing revealed the following results:

> Estradiol: Normal
> Progesterone: Normal
> Progesterone-estradiol ratio: Low
> Testosterone: Low
> Dehydroepiandrosterone sulfate (DHEAS): Low
> Cortisol: Morning - Normal
>   Bedtime - High

Diagnosis

Estrogen dominance, deficiencies of progesterone, dehydroepiandrosterone (DHEA), and androgen, coronary artery disease, high levels of cholesterol and triglycerides, high blood pressure, obesity, adrenal dysfunction

☞ Treatment

- A combination of bioidentical hormones (progesterone 30 mg/mL, testosterone 0.3 mg/mL, and dehydroepiandrosterone [DHEA] 1.5 mg/mL) in a cream (1 mL to be applied to a thin-skinned area such as the inner arm or inner thigh at bedtime or 0.5 mL to be applied in the morning and 0.5 mL to a different thin-skinned area at bedtime) (see Chapter 6).

- Following the Mediterranean diet.

- Practicing yoga 3 times weekly (see Chapter 3).

- Scheduling a Bio-Touch session once weekly (see Chapter 7).

- Completing a handwork project (see Chapter 5).

- Keeping a diary of symptoms.

- Joining a TOPS (Take Off Pounds Sensibly) support group.

☞ Suggested reading

Lee JR, Zava D, Hopkins H. *What Your Doctor May Not Tell You About Breast Cancer: How Hormone Balance Can Save Your Life.* New York, NY: Warner Books, Inc; 2002.

Wilson JL. *Adrenal Fatigue: The 21st Century Stress Syndrome.* Petaluma, Calif: Smart Publications; 2001. Web site: www.adrenalfatigue.org.

Spangle L. *Life Is Hard, Food Is Easy: The 5-Step Plan To Overcome Emotional Eating and Lose Weight on Any Diet.* Washington, DC: LifeLine Press; 2003.

☞ *Internet resources*

www.americanheart.org — A link to information about women and heart disease.

www.salivatest.com — A link to ZRT Laboratory, which provides saliva testing.

www.adrenalfatigue.org — A link to a Web site offering information about adrenal fatigue.

www.oldwayspt.org/pyramids — A link to a Web site offering information about the Mediterranean diet.

www.tops.org — TOPS (Take Off Pounds Sensibly) support group.

Follow Up

At her 2-month follow-up visit, BB had noted a marked decrease in the occurrence of hot flashes and an improvement in cognition, mood, and energy level. She had experienced no adverse effects from treatment with bioidentical hormone replacement therapy (BHRT). The results of saliva testing indicated that all hormone values were in the normal range.

Case 3. Replacing Self-Neglect with Self-Esteem

CC, a 65-year-old woman, presented with several health concerns. She stated that she had not been examined by a physician in years because she had no health insurance, but she had recently decided that she needed medical evaluation. She said that she experienced abdominal pain and chest pain 2 to 3 times per week. The episodes of pain would last for several hours but were not severe enough to cause her to stop her activities. She had gained more than 50 pounds over the last several years. CC complained of diarrhea that alternated with constipation, fatigue, weakness, poor sleep, joint pain, shortness of breath, and headaches.

At the time of her evaluation, CC was being treated with no medication. She had suffered from pneumonia 5 years earlier. Many years ago, she had undergone back surgery to treat a herniated disk. Her gallbladder had been removed, and she had undergone hysterectomy (both ovaries were preserved). She had experienced 4 normal pregnancies with normal deliveries. Both of her parents had died of a heart attack, and a sibling had high blood pressure.

CC lived with her spouse and adopted grandchild. She did not work outside the home. She did not drink alcohol or smoke. Her diet was high in meat, carbohydrates, and fats. She rarely prepared fruits and vegetables because of her family's food preferences. She did not exercise and spent most of her leisure time watching television as much as 4 to 5 hours per day. She said that her stress level was high because she was raising her grandchild.

CC was obese and had high blood pressure. She underwent an electrocardiogram, the results of which were in the normal range. She declined testing to determine her levels of various hormones. Serum testing revealed the following results:

> Total cholesterol: High
> Triglycerides: High
> Glucose: High normal
> Insulin: High
> Thyroid hormones: Normal

Diagnosis
Metabolic syndrome, fatigue, obesity, high total cholesterol level, high levels of triglycerides, high blood pressure, chest pain, joint pain, irritable bowel syndrome

☞ Treatment
- Fish oil[1] (3 g daily in capsule form).

- Guggul extract to improve the levels of triglycerides and cholesterol and enhance thyroid function.[2,3]

- Coenzyme Q_{10} for cardiovascular protection.[4,5]

- Enalapril maleate (Vasotec) to treat high blood pressure.

- Reducing the consumption of foods with a high glycemic index.

- Increasing the consumption of fruits and vegetables.

- Following the Mediterranean diet.

- Drinking water instead of sugared caffeinated beverages.

- Beginning an aerobic exercise program of walking 4 to 5 days per week.

- Practicing yoga learned via video instruction 1 to 3 times weekly (see Chapter 3).

- Completing a handwork project (see Chapter 5).

- Scheduling a Bio-Touch session once weekly (see Chapter 7).

☞ Cinematherapy
- *What's Cooking* (2000)

- *Babette's Feast*

☞ Suggested reading

Williamson M. *A Woman's Worth*. New York, NY: Random House; 1993.

Myss CM. *Anatomy of the Spirit: The Seven Stages of Power and Healing*. New York, NY: Three Rivers Press; 1996.

Ban Breathnach S. *Romancing the Ordinary: A Year of Simple Splendor*. New York, NY: Simple Abundance Press/Scribner; 2002. — A source of inspirational thoughts and ideas for self-care.

☞ Internet resource:

www.oldwayspt.org/pyramids — A link to a Web site offering information about the Mediterranean diet.

Follow Up

At her 4-month follow-up visit, CC reported no further chest pain or abdominal pain. She stated that she had more energy and a renewed sense of vitality. She had changed her diet dramatically to include fresh fruits and vegetables, and she ate meat and high-fat foods only occasionally. She stated that her husband had refused to change his eating habits, so she was preparing Mediterranean diet selections for herself and traditional Southern foods for her husband (an arrangement that was working well). She was exercising 5 days per week and had lost 20 pounds. Repeat laboratory testing indicated that her total cholesterol level had decreased by 100 points and her triglyceride levels by 200 points.

Secondary Follow Up

At her 6-month follow-up visit, CC had lost an additional 13 pounds. Her blood pressure was in the low-normal range, but she had noted an occasional feeling of light-headedness, so her dosage of Vasotec (which controls high blood pressure) was decreased. She had included the use of free weights in her exercise program. Her self-esteem had improved markedly. She had purchased new clothes for the first time in years and was pleased with her new hairstyle. Repeat laboratory testing revealed that her levels of glucose and insulin were within the normal range.

Discussion

As stated in Case 11 of Appendix B, metabolic syndrome is very common (and frequently misdiagnosed) in women. It is a combination of at least 3 or more of the following traits: high blood pressure (a value greater than 130/85), a high level of triglycerides (greater than or equal to 150 mg/dl) in the blood, a low level (less than or equal to 50 mg/dl) of HDL, a high fasting plasma glucose level (greater than or equal to 110), or abdominal obesity (a waist circumference of 35 inches or greater). It can contribute to the development of heart disease and diabetes. The symptoms of metabolic syndrome can be alleviated in part by changes in diet and lifestyle.

At the time of her initial appointment, CC's health had markedly declined. She was experiencing a constellation of symptoms that I believe were directly related to her diet, sedentary lifestyle, stress, and low self-esteem. The health-related improvement that she experienced by changing or controlling those factors suggests that like CC, other women can greatly improve their health and undo the effects of self-neglect. Many patients do not have to immediately begin a regimen of drug therapy to relieve symptoms caused by stress and a sedentary lifestyle. They can often improve their health by implementing affordable, practical changes in diet and exercise.

References

1. Covington MB. Omega-3 fatty acids. *Am Fam Physician.* 2004;70(1):133-140.

2. Urizar NL, Liverman AB, Dodds DT, et al. A natural product that lowers cholesterol as an antagonist ligand for the FXR. *Science.* 2002;296(5573):1703-1706.

3. Panda S, Kar A. Gugulu (Commiphora mukul) induces triiodothyronine production: possible involvement of lipid peroxidation. *Life Sci.* 1999;65(12):PL137-PL 141.

4. Langsjoen PH, Langsjoen AM. Coenzyme Q10 in cardiovascular disease with emphasis on heart failure and ischemia reperfusion. *Asia Pacific Heart J.* 1998;7(3):160-168.

5. Langsjoen PH, Langsjoen AM. Overview of the use of CoQ10 in cardiovascular disease. *Biofactors.* 1999;9(2-4):273-284.

Case 4. The Hazards of Being Home Alone

DD, a female patient in her mid-60s, suffered from multiple chronic medical problems that were treated with a variety of prescribed drugs. She experienced recurrent infections and often arrived in a wheelchair for her appointments. DD lived a reclusive lifestyle; she ventured away from home only to keep appointments with her physicians. She could be witty and engaging with the office staff, but she seemed sad and withdrawn most of the time. She confided that she had been unable to forgive herself for having broken a promise that she had made to herself.

DD's childhood was profoundly and negatively affected by the divorce of her parents. When she married and had children, she vowed that she would never divorce her husband. She remained with him even though their marriage was severely troubled, but when his abuse endangered her children, she left the marriage. She then sentenced herself to a life of isolation and misery for what she thought of as her failure. Guilt was her most consistent feeling.

☞ Treatment

I treated DD's many medical problems with appropriate therapies, but I knew that her emotional state contributed greatly to her lack of well-being. I prescribed the following therapy to address her feelings of guilt and sadness:

- Practicing "bed top" yoga taught via video or audio instruction (see Chapter 3).

- Dickman C. *Bed Top Yoga* [video]. Studio name not available; 1999.

- Dickman C. *Bed Top Yoga*. 1st edition [audio cassette]. Yoga Enterprises; 1997.

- Scheduling a Bio-Touch session once weekly (see chapter 7).

- Completing a handwork project (see Chapter 5).

- Volunteering in the community 4 hours weekly.

☞ Cinematherapy
- *Unbreakable*

- *The Terminal*

☞ Suggested reading
Forward S, Frazier D. *Emotional Blackmail: When the People in Your Life Use Fear, Obligation, and Guilt to Manipulate You*. New York, NY: Harper Audio; 1997.

Borysenko J. *Guilt Is the Teacher, Love Is the Lesson*. New York, NY: Warner Books; 1990.

Peck MS. *A Bed By the Window: A Novel of Mystery and Redemption*. New York, NY: Bantam Books; 1991.

Follow Up
When DD asked how she could improve her immune system to prevent recurrent infections, I suggested that she increase the number and variety of her social interactions and consider Bio-Touch treatment. She had stated that she rarely received a caring type of touch. DD then agreed with some skepticism to undergo a weekly Bio-Touch session.

After she had followed the suggestions listed above for 4 to 5 months, DD began to warily venture out on a few excursions other than those involving appointments with her doctors. She had begun to come alive and to display her personality and charm. She felt better and had experienced no serious infection. When I last saw her, she had made several friends. She was beginning to forgive herself and to start living again.

Discussion

Women debilitated by illness often isolate themselves to reduce the likelihood of contracting an infection, but research reveals that people with fewer social interactions are more vulnerable to infectious illnesses.[1] A research study showed that the common cold was less likely to develop in subjects who experienced multiple social interactions with people in various age groups.[2] Negative emotions and social isolation cause psychologic stress that can depress immune system function. As a result, chronic illnesses can worsen, and the vulnerability to infection increases.[3] Socially isolated women are more likely to experience frequent thoughts about negative past experiences than are socially active women. I have observed that patients who help others through volunteer work are less focused and obsessed with their own problems, at least for a while. By connecting with others instead of withdrawing, women (even those with a chronic illness) can improve their health and sense of well-being.

References

1. Uchino BN, Cacioppo JT, Kiecolt-Glaser JK. The relationship between social support and physiological processes: a review with emphasis on underlying mechanisms and implications for health. *Psychol Bull.* 1996;119(3):488-531.

2. Cohen S, Doyle WJ, Skoner DP, Rabin BS, Gwaltney JM Jr. Social ties and susceptibility to the common cold. *JAMA.* 1997;277(24):1940-1944.

3. Kiecolt-Glaser JK, McGuire L, Robles TF, Glaser R. Psychoneuroimmunology: psychological influences on immune function and health. *J Consult Clin Psychol.* 2002;70(3):537-547.

Case 5. The Power of Forgiveness

EE, a 68-year-old female patient, complained of an increase in her blood pressure despite compliance with her medication regimen. She was also experiencing tension headaches and disturbed sleep. The results of her physical examination and laboratory tests revealed no cause for concern. I recommended an increase in the dosage of the medication used to manage her hypertension and suggested that she continue to keep a diary of fluctuations in her blood pressure.

Follow Up

At the time of her 4-week follow-up appointment, EE's symptoms had not improved, and her blood pressure diary showed several episodes of hypertension. I asked her if she had been stressed or worried, and she seemed reluctant to respond. I revised her treatment regimen. Her next evaluation revealed continued high blood pressure in addition to frequent tension headaches and disturbed sleep. Physical examination showed no changes in her health status. I again asked EE if she had been under emotional stress, and she reluctantly nodded her head. She then said that she had not seen her granddaughter, whom she missed terribly, in several months. She explained that her son had died, and her daughter-in-law had had his body cremated. According to EE's belief system, cremation was an unthinkable act. She responded by severing ties with her daughter-in-law and then with her granddaughter. EE began to speak more forcefully about the unforgivable act of cremation. I suggested that her feelings about both her son's death and the estrangement from his family might be related to her symptoms, and I asked her to meet with a counselor on staff. EE agreed, and over the next few months her physical symptoms diminished as she began the inner work of forgiveness and acceptance.

☞ *Cinematherapy:*
- *Terms of Endearment*

- *Steel Magnolias*

☞ *Suggested reading:*
Myss CM. *Anatomy of the Spirit: The Seven Stages of Power and Healing.* New York, NY: Three Rivers Press; 1996.

Borysenko J. *Guilt Is the Teacher, Love Is the Lesson.* New York, NY: Warner Books; 1990.

Kingsolver B, Robertson D. *The Poisonwood Bible: A Novel.* New York, NY : HarperFlamingo; 1998.

Case 6. Caregiver Stress
FF, a 68-year-old female patient, came to my office for her annual wellness checkup. She appeared weary and stressed. During the visit, I asked about her relationships and living circumstances. She stated that she was the sole caregiver for her husband, a war veteran who suffered from emotional and physical problems caused by age-related diseases and prolonged internment in a prisoner-of-war camp decades ago. She said that they had had a very brief courtship and had quickly married before he was sent overseas. When he returned from the war several years later, he was markedly changed, but she felt that it was her duty to remain with him.

FF stated that her husband was prone to angry outbursts and fits of rage and that he was paranoid. Over the years, he had alienated friends and family. FF's life was spent caring for his physical and emotional needs. He frequently awakened her during the night, and she stated that her only time of peace was about 5:00 AM, when he typically slept for 30 to 45 minutes. She spent that time reading and praying. She ventured out on brief excursions to the hair salon or grocery store, but if she did not return within a specified period of time, her husband reacted angrily. Because he did not like her talking to friends on the phone, she had little social contact and was not able to maintain friendships.

FF had thought about obtaining home health care that would provide some assistance and relief, but her husband forbade this and stated that he would not allow strangers in the house. Clearly the recurring themes in her relationship and daily activities were fear, obligation, and guilt (see Chapter 2). FF was extremely resistant to placing her husband in a veterans healthcare facility. I expressed my concern about her situation and her health. I emphasized that living under prolonged chronic psychologic stress placed her at high risk for a heart attack.

☞ Treatment
- Practicing yoga 1 to 3 times weekly (see Chapter 3).

- Scheduling a Bio-Touch session once weekly (see Chapter 7).

- Completing a handwork project (see Chapter 5).

☞ Cinematherapy
- *Paradise Road* (1997)

☞ Suggested reading
Estes, Pinkola C. *Women Who Run with the Wolves: Myths and Stories of the Wild Woman Archetype.* New York, NY: Ballantine Books; 1995.

Borysenko J. *Guilt Is the Teacher, Love Is the Lesson.* New York, NY: Warner Books; 1990.

Cameron A. *Daughters of Copper Woman.* Vancouver, BC: Press Gang Publishers; 1981.

Ban Breathnach S. *Simple Abundance: A Daybook of Comfort and Joy.* New York, NY: Warner Books; 1995.

Follow Up

FF returned several months later and demanded to see what she referred to as my crystal ball. She appeared years younger, more vibrant, and relaxed. She related that shortly after her appointment with me, she had suffered a massive heart attack while she was shoveling snow in her driveway. The neighbors had called 911 to summon help. FF had undergone emergency surgery, after which she suffered shock and episodes of irregular heartbeat. She stated that the members of the medical team were baffled by her heart attack because she had no traditional risk factors (diabetes, high blood pressure, high levels of cholesterol and triglycerides, a history of smoking, obesity) for heart disease.

During FF's hospitalization, arrangements were made for her husband's immediate admission to a veterans healthcare facility. When FF recovered and was discharged from the hospital, she decided that her husband should remain in that residence because he would receive excellent medical care and his needs would be provided for. She occasionally brought him home for a few brief visits but had been very firm in setting limits to the duration of his stay and the schedule for his return to the healthcare facility.

Case 7. A Cure for Painful Sex

GG, a 69-year-old female patient, presented with complaints of extreme pain that occurred during sexual activity. She had been treated with tamoxifen for 5 years after having undergone a radical mastectomy as treatment for breast cancer. She had been advised that she should never receive treatment with any type of hormone.

To relieve her discomfort, GG had treated herself with multiple nonhormonal and herbal options. All were ineffective. Physical examination revealed severe atrophy of the vulva and vagina. In some areas, the vaginal and vulvar skin was thin and fine and bled with light pressure. GG had just entered a new relationship after having been divorced for many years, and she wanted to enjoy sexual activity. Saliva testing revealed the following ranges of the hormones listed below:

> Estradiol: Low
> Estrone: Normal
> Estriol: Low
> Progesterone-estradiol ratio: Low
> Testosterone: Normal
> Dehydroepiandrosterone sulfate (DHEAS): Normal
> Cortisol: Morning - Normal
> Evening - High

☞ Treatment

To relieve GG's symptoms, I prescribed the following treatment:

- Estriol vaginal suppositories 1 mg (1 suppository to be inserted vaginally each night for 3 nights, then 2 to 3 nights per week) (see Chapter 6).

- Bioidentical progesterone cream 20 mg/mL (1 mL to be applied at bedtime to a thin-skinned area such as the inner arm or inner thigh) (see Chapter 6).

☞ Cinematherapy
- *Something's Gotta Give*

☞ Suggested reading
Lee JR, Zava D, Hopkins H. *What Your Doctor May Not Tell You About Breast Cancer: How Hormone Balance Can Save Your Life*. New York, NY: Warner Books, Inc; 2002.

Holstein LL. *How to Have Magnificent Sex : The 7 Dimensions of a Vital Sexual Connection.* New York, NY: Harmony Books; 2001.

☞ *Internet resource:*
www.aasect.org — American Association of Sex Educators, Counselors, and Therapists.

Follow Up

Within 4 weeks, GG reported significant symptom relief from the pain that had occurred during sexual activity. However, she had also noted diminished sexual arousal and orgasm, so I prescribed compounded sildenafil (Viagra) 2% cream with optional flavoring, such as chocolate or pina colada, to be used as needed (a pea-size amount was to be placed on the clitoral area 20 to 30 minutes before sexual activity). As mentioned in Case 10 of Appendix B, an increase in the blood flow to the genitals is thought to trigger sexual responsiveness. In my clinical experience, about 40% of women who complain of diminished libido benefit to some degree from this treatment, but others find it ineffective or experience unpleasant sensations when the cream is applied. Those differences in the response to therapy may be due to the variability and complexity of female sexual arousal and response patterns. GG later reported a positive response to treatment with this compounded medication.

Discussion

Female sexual dysfunction includes disorders of desire, arousal, or orgasm; painful intercourse; and vaginismus (an involuntary contraction of the muscles in the genital area when penetration is attempted). Older women experience sexual problems, but many physicians are reluctant to ask about that aspect of a patient's life. They often assume that single older women are not sexually active.

Asking a patient questions about her sexual function should be part of a complete patient assessment. I have found that patients often want to discuss their sexual concerns with their physician. Sexual problems can significantly affect a woman's quality of life and stress level. Some women benefit from working with a sex therapist who is affiliated with a physician. Sex therapists diagnose and treat sexual disorders and provide education for patients. They are skilled in helping women resolve the trauma of past physical or sexual abuse and in counseling couples who are experiencing marital discord. They also teach specific skills that promote sexual desire and lessen performance anxiety.

Case 8. Overcoming Tragedy and Loss

HH, a 71-year-old female patient, was alone in the world. She was widowed and had no children. Her parents and sister were deceased. She had several chronic illnesses (heart disease, diabetes, arthritis, chronic knee pain) that caused physical discomfort and limited her lifestyle. During her appointments, however, she never complained about her suffering. She was always cheerful, inquisitive, and nurturing and would light up the room with her presence. Seeing her name on the patient schedule always brightened my day.

During one of HH's frequent hospitalizations, I met several of her many visitors. Most of them were neighbors; young couples who described HH as the "grandmother of the neighborhood." She cooked for them, played games with their children, cared for their pets, and was always ready to listen to their problems. HH later shared her personal story with me. The elder of 2 Jewish sisters, she was born before World War II in Germany. Her father, who was in the German military, died in combat during the war. One night near the end of the war, HH and her sister, who were both teenagers, were unexpectedly accosted by German authorities and were taken to a nearby hospital. There they underwent a surgical procedure that was listed officially as appendectomy, although neither girl had exhibited the signs of appendicitis or any other disease before surgery.

There was great social and economic upheaval in Germany as the war ended, and at the age of 17 years, HH was separated from her mother and sister. She soon secured a job that was related to the US military occupation. She met, fell in love with, and married an American serviceman with whom she came to the United States. She and her husband wanted a family, but HH was unable to conceive. She was evaluated by several specialists, who determined that both fallopian tubes had been removed, apparently during the surgical procedure that HH had undergone during the war. A victim of forced sterilization in Nazi Germany, HH was infertile. When her husband received that news, he left her.

HH later married another man who accepted her infertility, and they had a loving marriage until he died. When the Berlin Wall was torn down in 1989, HH was shocked and delighted to receive a letter from her sister, with whom she immediately arranged a reunion. Although they had been separated for more than 40 years, HH and her sister immediately reconnected emotionally. I thought that HH certainly had a right to be bitter, angry, and resentful, but she was just the opposite. Her grace in not dwelling on personal injustice and circumstances was a spiritually powerful force that was very inspiring.

☞ *Cinematherapy:*
- *Out of Rosenheim* (1987), also titled (Bagdad Café) (1988)

- *The Color Purple*

Discussion

Like HH, many women who have lived through devastating circumstances and tragic events move ahead to exhibit a passion for living and a heightened ability to connect with others in a caring, nurturing manner. Viktor E. Frankl, a concentration camp survivor and a psychiatrist, has written about the profound resilience of the human spirit in his book *Man's Search for Ultimate Meaning* (New York, NY: Fine Communications, 2002).

Case 9. Making the Right Choice

VV, a 75-year-old female patient, was concerned about using hormone replacement therapy (HRT) to relieve the symptoms of menopause. She had been treated with conjugated equine estrogens (Premarin) for many years. When she attempted to stop that treatment, she experienced severe hot flashes, night sweats, headaches, a craving for sugar, moodiness, and palpitations. If she resumed treatment with Premarin, those symptoms improved, but VV was concerned about the long-term effects of synthetic hormones and preferred therapy with bioidentical hormone replacement therapy (BHRT).

At the time of her appointment, VV had resumed treatment with Premarin. She also took a daily calcium supplement, a multivitamin, and additional vitamin E, C, and B complex. She suffered from no chronic illnesses but had undergone hysterectomy and the removal of both ovaries. She had experienced 1 normal pregnancy with an uneventful delivery.

VV's mother had died of heart disease, and her father had died of a stroke. She was widowed and lived alone. She had a college education and was an active volunteer in her community. She ate a low-fat diet and did not drink caffeinated beverages. She did not smoke. She drank 2 glasses of wine weekly. VV exercised by following a walking program. She admitted to being under emotional stress in a serious relationship; she was being pressured to consider marriage but was concerned about her prospective husband's health. VV had taken care of a chronically ill spouse for several years and was hesitant to resume that role. In addition, there was conflict among extended family members about the relationship.

VV's weight was within the normal range for her height. Atrophy of the vulva and vagina was noted during physical examination. Serum and saliva testing revealed the following results:

Serum testing (range)
Thyroid hormones: Normal

Saliva testing (range)
Estradiol: Normal
Progesterone: Normal
Progesterone-estradiol ratio: Slightly low
Testosterone: Low
Dehydroepiandrosterone sulfate (DHEAS): Low
Cortisol: Morning - Normal
Noon - High
Evening - High
Bedtime - High

Diagnosis
Effects of menopause, stress, deficiencies of androgens and progesterone, adrenal dysfunction

☞ Treatment
- A cream containing the following bioidentical hormones: progesterone 30 mg/mL, testosterone 0.3 mg/mL, Tri-Est (80% estriol, 10% estradiol, and 10% estrone) 0.25 mg/mL, and dehydroepiandrosterone (DHEA) 1.5 mg/mL (1 mL to be applied at bedtime to a thin-skinned area

such as the inner thigh or the inner arm) (see Chapter 6).

- Estriol vaginal suppositories 1 mg (1 vaginal suppository at bedtime for 3 nights, then 1 suppository 2 to 3 times weekly at bedtime) (see Chapter 6).

- Practicing yoga 1 to 3 times weekly (see Chapter 3) .

- Scheduling a Bio-Touch session once weekly (see Chapter 7).

- Completing a handwork project (see Chapter 5).

☞ Cinematherapy
- *Fried Green Tomatoes*

- *Cocoon*

- *Terms of Endearment*

☞ Suggested reading
Northrup C. *The Wisdom of Menopause: Creating Physical and Emotional Health and Healing During the Change.* New York, NY: Bantam Books; 2001.

Forward S, Frazier D. *Emotional Blackmail: When the People in Your Life Use Fear, Obligation, and Guilt to Manipulate You.* New York, NY: Harper Audio; 1997.

Follow Up
At her 8-week follow-up visit, VV stated that some of her symptoms had improved but she was continuing to experience palpitations, sometimes with associated fatigue and chest tightness. Repeat saliva testing showed that VV's hormone profile was in the normal range except for a slightly low level of progesterone. She attributed her symptoms to a hormone imbalance; however, because of her age and the symptoms that she reported, further evaluation of her heart was important. The results of stress testing, Holter monitor recordings, and echocardio-

graphy revealed cardiac problems, and VV was referred to a cardiologist for treatment.

Discussion

Older women are not exempt from stressful relationships and turmoil in life. Our popular cultural images do not often include courting among the elderly, which is a real dilemma for many women. Because most US women live longer than their male counterparts,[1] they often become the primary caregiver for an ill spouse. The stress of that role can be an emotional roller coaster. Caregivers are often given responsibility and authority by immediate and extended family who do not want to assume duties and obligations. Those same family members, however, may be quick to criticize the decisions made by the primary caregiver. In addition, months or years may pass before many caregivers are granted the respite of a vacation or even an afternoon off. Such unrelenting stress is detrimental to physical and emotional health. For women in their 70s, whose knowledge has been gained from experience, making a decision about marriage may be even more stressful than it is for younger women.

Reference

1. Arias E. United States Life Tables, 2001. Natl Vital Stat Rep. 2004;52(14):1-38. Also available at: http://www.cdc.gov/nchs/data/nvsr/nvsr52/nvsr52_14.pdf. Accessed June 22, 2004.

Case 10. Early Diagnosis, Early Treatment

JJ, a 76-year-old female patient, was concerned about menopausal symptoms. She had suffered from noninsulin-dependent diabetes for many years and also had high blood pressure and hypothyroidism. She had stopped taking conjugated equine estrogens (Premarin) 6 months earlier. Since that time, she had experienced hot flashes, vaginal dryness, irritable mood, fatigue, short-term memory problems, and a decreased ability to concentrate on cognitive (mental) tasks.

At the time of her appointment, JJ was being treated with lisinopril (Zestril) to control high blood pressure, metformin hydrochloride (Glucophage) to manage diabetes, and levothyroxine sodium (Synthroid) to treat hypothyroidism. She also took a daily multivitamin and a daily calcium supplement. She declined treatment with lipid-lowering drugs or aspirin. She had undergone heart bypass surgery several years earlier, as well as hysterectomy and the removal of both ovaries when she was in her 40s.

JJ, who had a college degree, lived with her spouse. She ate a low-fat diet and exercised at a health club several times weekly. She volunteered in her community several times weekly. She did not smoke or drink alcohol, and she described her relationship with her husband and children as good.

JJ's weight was normal for her height. The results of the Beck Depression Inventory indicated mild-to-moderate depression. Her score on the Folstein Mini Mental Status Examination was within the normal range. Serum and saliva testing revealed the following results:

Serum testing (range)
> Thyroid hormones: Normal
> Complete blood count: Normal
> Basic metabolic panel: Normal
> Lipid levels: Normal

Saliva testing (range)
> Estradiol: Normal
> Progesterone: Normal
> Progesterone-estradiol ratio: Low
> Testosterone: Low

Dehydroepiandrosterone sulfate (DHEAS): Low
Cortisol: Morning - Low
        Noon - Low
        Evening - Low
        Bedtime - Low

Diagnosis

Estrogen dominance; deficiency of progesterone, dehydroepiandrosterone (DHEA), and androgen; adrenal exhaustion; diabetes; high blood pressure; heart disease; depression

☙ *Treatment*

- A cream containing the following bioidentical hormones: progesterone 20 mg/mL, bioidentical testosterone 0.3 mg/mL, and DHEA 1.5 mg/mL (1 mL to be applied at bedtime to a thin-skinned area such as the inner arm or inner thigh) (see Chapter 6).

- Sertraline (Zoloft) as antidepressant therapy.

Follow Up

At her 8-week follow-up visit, JJ said that the suggested treatment had produced some relief from hot flashes but that problems with her short-term memory had continued. Her mood had improved slightly and her fatigue had diminished somewhat, probably as a result of treatment with Zoloft and bioidentical hormone replacement therapy (BHRT). Follow-up saliva testing showed that her levels of estradiol, progesterone, testosterone, and DHEAS were in the normal range but that her levels of cortisol remained below normal. Her score on the Folstein Mini Mental Status Examination had decreased by several points, and I recommended further neurologic testing. The results confirmed early dementia, and treatment was initiated.

Discussion

Women are more likely than men to be diagnosed with dementia, including Alzheimer's disease.[1] Early diagnosis is critical, because current medical therapies have been shown to slow the progression of dementia if treatment is initiated early in the course of the disease. Unfortunately, many women and their family members deny or conceal the signs of dementia, and diagnosis is made when the disease has progressed.

Because of JJ's symptoms and her depression, I had prescribed a trial of antidepressant medication after her first examination. Although depression is most often diagnosed in women who range in age from 20 to 50 years,[1] elderly women are also at risk. Screening for depression should be a part of the routine evaluation of women who have heart disease. Like JJ, they are more at risk for depression than are men.

Internet resource:

www.alz.org — Alzheimer's Association, telephone: 800-272-3900

Reference

1. Carlson KJ, Eisenstat SA, Ziporyn TD. *The New Harvard Guide to Women's Health*. Cambridge, Mass: Harvard University Press; 2004.

Case 11. Anniversaries and Emotional Trauma

KK, a female patient in her 70s, had been in my care for several years. She had high blood pressure but no other medical problems. Each spring, her blood pressure would become uncontrollable, and her husband would bring her to the office for evaluation. After several weeks and several urgent office visits during which KK was treated for high blood pressure, standard medications for that disorder would again become effective. During the third year of this pattern, I asked KK whether a stressful "anniversary date" occurred during spring. She nodded her head but stated the event was too terrible to talk about.

Over the next few visits, KK explained that she had first become pregnant when she was in her early 20s. She was unmarried and could not afford to care for a child, so she made the difficult decision to give up her baby for adoption. Fifty years later, the memory of that experience was powerful enough to exert a profound physical effect on KK as her first child's birthday approached. She said that she felt both guilt and grief when she thought about having given up her baby. She confided that she had never shared that secret with anyone, including her husband and other children. Each year at the time of her first child's birthday, KK's feelings and thoughts about that pregnancy and the relinquishment of her child became more intense.

☞ *Treatment*
- Referral to a psychotherapist to address KK's ongoing grief and the trauma related to her experience as a birth mother.

- Referral to a therapist for treatment with eye movement desensitization and reprocessing (EMDR). As stated in Case 3 of Appendix B, EMDR therapy can eliminate or greatly decrease the emotional distress that is related to memories of traumatic events, even if they occurred years ago. I have found that EMDR can help victims of past trauma to reclaim their lost sense of self. During EMDR therapy, the patient recalls a past or present traumatic experience in brief episodes while performing a series of eye movements or focusing on an external stimulus such as auditory tones or tapping. After a rest period, the patient associates a positive thought with the memory of the unpleasant event.

☞ Suggested reading

Estes, Pinkola C. *Women Who Run with the Wolves: Myths and Stories of the Wild Woman Archetype.* New York, NY: Ballantine Books; 1995.

Soll J, Buterbaugh KW. *Adoption Healing: A Path to Recovery for Mothers Who Lost Children to Adoption.* New York, NY: Adoption Crossroads; 2003.

☞ Internet resource

www.emdr.org — EMDR Institute, Inc — Information on eye movement desensitization and reprocessing (EMDR)

Follow Up

KK decided to tell her husband and her other children about having arranged the adoption of her first baby. She also joined a support group for birthmothers in her area. By connecting with other women who had had similar experiences and felt similar emotions, she received much-needed psychosocial support and validation of her feelings. As KK began to consciously and deliberately address her feelings about this remote traumatic event, her blood pressure fluctuations diminished.

Discussion

I frequently ask women whose physical symptoms cannot be medically explained whether the anniversary date of a past traumatic event coincides with their illness. Research reveals a strong connection between the mind and the body, and women are more susceptible than are men to intrusive thoughts about negative experiences. When a woman begins thinking and deeply reflecting, she experiences an increase in blood pressure, heart rate, and cortisol release.[1,2]

Some patients with a medically unexplained symptom may not be aware of an anniversary date that is associated with their illness. When questioned, however, they often remember a past event that coincides with the season or date of symptom onset. Nondrug therapies such as EMDR, participation in a support group, or psychotherapy may assist women in overcoming repeated episodes of physical symptoms that have an emotional cause.

References

1. Baum A, Cohen L, Hall M. Control and intrusive memories as possible determinants of chronic stress. *Psychosom Med.* 1993;55(3):274-286.

2. Elenkov IJ, Chrousos GP. Stress, cytokine patterns and susceptibility to disease. *Baillieres Best Pract Res Clin Endocrinol Metab.* 1999;13(4):583-595.

Case 12. Writing Woes

LL, an 80-year-old female patient with heart disease, exhibited a familial tremor in her hands. Numerous medications were ineffective in controlling the tremor. LL always seemed to be frowning. During each visit, she emphasized how horrible the tremor was and asked whether new treatments for such disorders had become available. Eventually, I referred LL to a nationally known neurologist, who was unable to help her. She continued to focus on this sole symptom during every medical appointment and her life in general.

LL was a retired professional in the financial field and had enjoyed a highly successful career. She had never married and had no children. She had undergone cardiac bypass surgery several years earlier. Her parents and siblings were deceased. LL was extremely bothered by her difficulty in writing a check, balancing her bank statements, and writing letters of personal correspondence. She was so embarrassed about her tremor that she had stopped attending church and had dropped out of her bridge group, which had been her only social interactions.

☞ Treatment

- A new focus. I recommended that LL change her focus from the physical to the spiritual, which is a normal transition into the third phase of the feminine life cycle (see Chapter 2). Although LL was unable to write, she had many gifts that she was not using. I suggested that by helping others and accepting her limitations, she would begin to appreciate her own life each day. She might also be alert for technical devices that would compensate for some restrictions. We specifically discussed her hiring an assistant to help with writing and other tasks that required fine motor skills. I also recommended that she select a cause to support as a volunteer. She chose the local animal shelter because she felt that the animals there would not judge her.

☞ Cinematherapy

- *Driving Miss Daisy*

- *Finding Forrester*

- *Lost in Translation*

☞ Internet resource

www.ivaa.org — International Virtual Assistants Association — A Web site that provides virtual assistants.

Follow Up

At her 8-week follow-up appointment, LL could not stop talking about her new assistant, a young woman who helped with banking and personal correspondence and who was also interested in finance. LL greatly enjoyed her mentoring role, and she appreciated having legible numbers in her personal banking system and a source of attractive handwritten letters. She looked forward to the social interactions with her assistant and with the animals at the shelter. She did not complain about her tremor again.

Index

244, 247-264, 268-287, 292-308, 315-323, 334-337, 339-345
   formulations of, 126, 142
   functions of, 104
   research and, 127-129
   symptoms of imbalance, 110

Pseudoseizures, case study, 207-210

Sandtray therapy, 74-78
   case studies, 76-77, 289-292

Sex drive, case studies, 277-281, 334-337

Sexual trauma, case studies, 76, 201-204, 211-215

Sleep disturbance, case studies, 193-197

Television viewing
   case studies, 188-197, 323-328
   women, 84-85

Testosterone
   case studies, 240-244, 247-253, 257-264, 277-281, 292-300, 320-323, 339-345
   formulations of, 126, 142
   function of, 104
   symptoms of imbalance of, 110-111

Thyroid hormone
   case studies, 223-228, 240-244, 257-264, 292-296, 304-308
   formulation of, 142
   function of, 107
   interaction with other hormones, 107-108

Touch
   animals and, 146-148
   humans and, 146, 148-158

Tri-Est
   case studies, 292-296, 339-342
   formulations of, 126, 142
   use of, 126

Uterine fibroids, case study, 300-304

Veterans
   gender and, 1, 9
   handwork and, 96-97
   post traumatic stress disorder and, 95
   sandtray therapy and, 75-78

Weight gain
   hormone imbalance and, 110-111, 124

Women's health
   lack of health insurance and, case studies, 264-266, 323-328
   principles of, 5-13
   research and, 2-3

Women's Health Initiative, 3-5, 120-121

Working women, 35-40

Xenohormones, 106-107

Yoga, 35, 40-47
   bedtop, 46-47
   benefits of, 40-46
   research and, 41-46

The Goddess Athena

Uncited References

Readers interested in obtaining more information about the goddess Athena and Greek mythology and literature may enjoy the following texts:

Godolphin FRB, ed. Borroum FR, ed. *Great Classical Myths*. New York, NY: Random House, Inc; 1964.

Bowra CM. *Landmarks in Greek Literature*. London, England: Weidenfeld & Nicolson; 1966.

Francisca AH. *People and Themes in Homer's Odyssey*. London, England: Thornton Methuen & Co LTD; 1970.

Rabinowitz NS, Richlin A, eds. *Feminist Theory and the Classics*. New York, NY: Routledge; 1993.

Lesky A. *A History of Greek Literature*. London, England: Methuen & Co Ltd; 1966.

Mascetti MD. *Athena: Goddess of War and Wisdom*. San Francisco, Calif: Chronicle Books; 1996.